Metabolic Confusion Diet

For Endomorph Women

Increase your metabolism with a 28 day meal plan to unlock the secrets of weight loss with proven easy-to-follow recipes

Laurie W. Lamb

Thank You For Reading!!

I hope you will enjoy reading it as much as I enjoyd writing it.

<u>Your support means the world to me!.</u>

If you will find value in this pages,

I kindly ask you to consider **leaving an honest review on Amazon.**

Your feedback not only helps me improve but also helps other readers discover this

Book.

Table of Contents

INTRODUCTION

Welcome to a trip that could change your life and health! If you are an endomorph lady who is having trouble with weight control, energy fluctuations, and the feeling that your metabolic system is constantly at odds with you, you've come to the perfect spot. This book, Metabolic Confusion Diet For Endomorph Women, was created with you in mind.

As an endomorph, your body's metabolism is slightly altered. Traditional dieting approaches may not be effective for you, leaving you disappointed and disheartened. You are not alone. Many women, like yourself, face this dilemma. I've had the luxury of working with countless endomorphs who have felt precisely the same way—trapped in a cycle of dieting and disappointment.

But here's some good news: change is possible. This book is intended to provide a personalised strategy to eating and living based on your own metabolic demands. You'll learn about the basics of metabolic confusion, an approach that can revitalise your metabolism, allowing your body to burn fat more effectively and keep you energised all day.

These pages provide more than simply recipes; they also serve as a thorough guide to understanding how your body reacts to various meals and eating patterns. We'll go over practical measures for tailoring your diet to your unique needs, including meal plans that are simple to follow and full of flavour.

Each recipe is designed to be both delicious and beneficial to your metabolic health. However, this book is much than just a collection of recipes. It's a supportive friend that recognises your unique journey and offers specific actions to help you reach your health objectives. Here, you'll learn from real women who have used these tactics to alter their lives. Their experiences will inspire and encourage you that success is attainable.

So, if you're ready to end the cycle of dissatisfaction and adopt a diet that works for your body, let's get started. Dive into the upcoming chapters and take the first step towards a healthier, more vibrant you. By following the ideas stated in this book, you will be able to take charge of your health and well-being.

Don't wait any longer—your new adventure begins right now.
Order your copy today and begin the journey to metabolic balance and
restored vitality.

What is The Metabolic Confusion Diet?

The Metabolic Confusion Diet is a flexible eating plan that tries to keep your metabolism guessing by varying your calorie intake on different days. Unlike standard diets, in which you consume the same number of calories every day, this technique alternates between high-calorie and low-calorie days. The aim is to prevent your metabolism from adjusting to a certain calorie level, which might result in weight reduction plateaus.

For example, you could eat more calories one day to fuel your body, then consume less calories the next day to allow your body to use stored fat as energy. This alternate rhythm is thought to keep your metabolism busy, which helps you burn calories more efficiently.

This diet does not impose tight food restrictions, making it more suitable to various lives and interests. The emphasis is on the timing and amount of calories consumed, rather than eliminating specific food groups. This flexibility can make the Metabolic Confusion Diet easier to stick to in the long run, allowing for indulgences without fully derailing your progress.

Endomorph women, who have a slower metabolism and a higher inclination to accumulate fat, may benefit from the Metabolic Confusion Diet in various ways. This diet may be especially successful because it tackles the specific metabolic problems that endomorphs encounter.

1. **Boosts Metabolic Rate:** Endomorphs frequently have a slow metabolism, which makes it difficult to lose weight. The Metabolic Confusion Diet promotes a more active metabolism by constantly altering your caloric intake, preventing your body from falling into a metabolic rut.

2. **Supports Fat Loss While Maintaining Muscle:** By including high-calorie days, the diet guarantees that your body has adequate energy to maintain lean muscle mass. This is especially important for endomorphs, who are prone to losing muscle while dieting, which can further reduce their metabolism.

3. **Reduces Diet Fatigue:** Adhering to a strict low-calorie diet can be both psychologically and physically demanding. The alternating high-calorie days provide a mental break, making it simpler to stick to your overall weight loss goals. This flexibility may also lower the danger of binge eating, which is typical among those on restricted diets.

4. **Tailored for Hormonal Balance:** Endomorph women may have hormonal abnormalities that cause weight gain, particularly around the hips and thighs. The Metabolic Confusion Diet's diverse approach can assist stabilise hormones by avoiding excessive caloric shortages,

which can disturb your body's hormonal equilibrium.

5. **Enhanced Energy Levels:** The diet's structure allows for periods of higher calorie consumption, which can aid in energy maintenance, particularly during workouts. Endomorphs who feel tired on typical low-calorie diets may benefit greatly from this.

How It's Different from Other Diets

The Metabolic Confusion Diet is distinguished from other diets by its unique approach to calorie consumption.

Here's how it varies from several popular diets:

1. **Consistency vs. Variability:** Traditional diets, such as calorie-restricted or low-carb diets, frequently need regular daily calorie intake or specific food limitations. In contrast, the Metabolic Confusion Diet emphasises variability. It does not force you to stick to a strict dietary regimen, but rather encourages you to be more flexible.

2. **No Food Group Elimination:** Unlike keto and paleo diets, which eliminate entire food groups, the Metabolic Confusion Diet does not compel you to forego your favourite foods. This makes it more sustainable and less restrictive, which can improve long-term adherence.

3. **Prevention of Metabolic Slowdown:** Many diets, particularly low-calorie ones, can cause metabolism to slow down as the body adjusts to the lower energy intake. The Metabolic Confusion Diet seeks to avoid this by regularly varying your calorie intake, keeping your metabolism on its toes.

4. **Psychological Flexibility:** Diets such as intermittent fasting or low-carb diets frequently contain strict regulations that might be difficult to follow. The Metabolic Confusion Diet, on the other hand, provides greater psychological flexibility, lowering the risk of diet fatigue or burnout.

Scientific Basis of Metabolic Confusion

The Metabolic Confusion Diet's scientific base is built on the concept of "metabolic adaptation." When you maintain a steady low-calorie diet, your body gradually adapts by lowering your metabolism to conserve energy, a process known as adaptive thermogenesis. This can make it more difficult to lose weight over time as your body grows more effective at burning fewer calories.

By altering your caloric intake with the Metabolic Confusion Diet, you hope to disturb this adaptive process. On high-calorie days, your body receives a metabolic boost, which speeds up calorie burning, whereas on low-calorie days, it digs into fat stores without experiencing the same level of metabolic slowing.

This strategy is also backed by the principle of "calorie cycling," which has been researched in numerous ways. According to research, periodic intervals of higher calorie consumption can counteract the metabolic decline that usually occurs with extended dieting. Furthermore, alternating calorie consumption may assist maintain lean muscle mass, which is essential for a healthy metabolism.

Endomorph Body Type

Features of the Endomorph Body Type

The endomorph body type is frequently distinguished by a naturally higher percentage of body fat, a larger frame, and a proclivity to retain fat more easily than other body types. Women with this physique may note that they have a soft, rounder appearance, with weight increase primarily in the hips, thighs, and tummy. This body type typically has a slower metabolism, which can make weight loss difficult.

Endomorphs typically have a bigger bone structure and may appear fuller, even when they are at a healthy weight. Their muscles may be strong, but they are frequently less defined due to the layer of fat that surrounds them. Endomorphs, unlike ectomorphs, who are naturally slim and struggle to acquire weight, or mesomorphs, who are more muscular and athletic, may struggle to achieve a lean appearance unless their diet and exercise routines are well managed.

Challenges and Strengths.

Challenges:

Endomorph women confront specific issues, including managing weight and body composition. Because of their slower metabolic rate, people may acquire weight more easily and lose weight more slowly, even with a balanced diet and frequent exercise. This proclivity to store fat can cause dissatisfaction and discouragement, especially when compared to people with different body types who may notice faster results.

Another problem is the body's inclination to retain water, which can lead to feelings of bloating and impede weight loss efforts. Furthermore, because endomorphs are prone to insulin resistance, they may be more sensitive to carbohydrates, implying that eating too many carbs can result in fat accumulation rather than energy use.

Strengths

Endomorph women have strengths that can help them achieve their health and fitness objectives. One key advantage is their inherent strength and power. Endomorphs can quickly gain muscle with proper training, which can enhance metabolism and aid in fat loss.

Endomorphs also have a high energy reserve, allowing them to work out for longer and more intensely. This resilience can be an asset in a workout plan designed to help you lose weight and improve your overall health. Furthermore, their naturally curves and larger forms are frequently praised in today's body-positive movement, which emphasises the attractiveness of various body shapes.

Importance of Tailored Diet Plans for Endomorphs

Given the endomorph body type's distinct metabolic characteristics, it is critical to design a diet plan that meets their special requirements. Endomorphs' bodies respond differently to macronutrients than other body types, therefore a one-size-fits-all strategy to dieting is rarely effective.

Endomorph women are often advised to consume a diet rich in protein and healthy fats, with a moderate to low carbohydrate intake. Protein is required not just for muscle maintenance and growth, but also for increased satiety, which can aid to prevent overeating. Healthy fats, like those found in avocados, almonds, and olive oil, can provide long-lasting energy and promote overall health.

Carbohydrate management is especially crucial. Endomorphs benefit from consuming complex carbs such as whole grains, vegetables, and legumes, while avoiding simple sugars and processed carbs, which can raise insulin levels and increase fat accumulation. The timing of carbohydrate consumption might also play a role; for example, eating more carbs earlier in the day or around training times can assist optimise energy levels and reduce fat growth.

Caloric intake should be carefully controlled, as even little excesses might cause weight gain in endomorphs. However, extreme calorie restriction should be avoided because it might impede metabolism and cause muscle loss, which is detrimental to long-term weight management.

Metabolism and Weight Loss for Endomorphic Women

Metabolism influences how endomorph women maintain their weight. Endomorphs often have a slower metabolic rate, therefore they burn fewer calories at rest than other body types. This makes it critical to focus on increasing metabolism through food and exercise.

Exercise: Strength training is an efficient approach to boost metabolism in endomorphs. Building lean muscle mass increases the quantity of calories burned at rest, which can assist offset the body's naturally slow metabolism. Incorporating resistance training into your normal workout program, with a focus on compound movements like squats, deadlifts, and presses, can be very useful.

Cardiovascular activity also plays a role, particularly high-intensity interval training (HIIT), which has been found to be more effective at fat loss than steady-state cardio. HIIT burns calories throughout the workout and can keep the metabolism up for hours afterward.

Diet: A diet rich in protein, healthy fats, and managed carbohydrate intake can improve metabolic health. Furthermore, eating smaller, more frequent meals throughout the day can help regulate blood sugar levels and prevent overeating, which is critical for weight management.

Lifestyle: Other important lifestyle aspects include getting enough sleep and managing stress. Lack of sleep and persistent stress can both have a bad impact on metabolism and lead to weight gain, particularly in endomorphs who are inclined to accumulating fat.

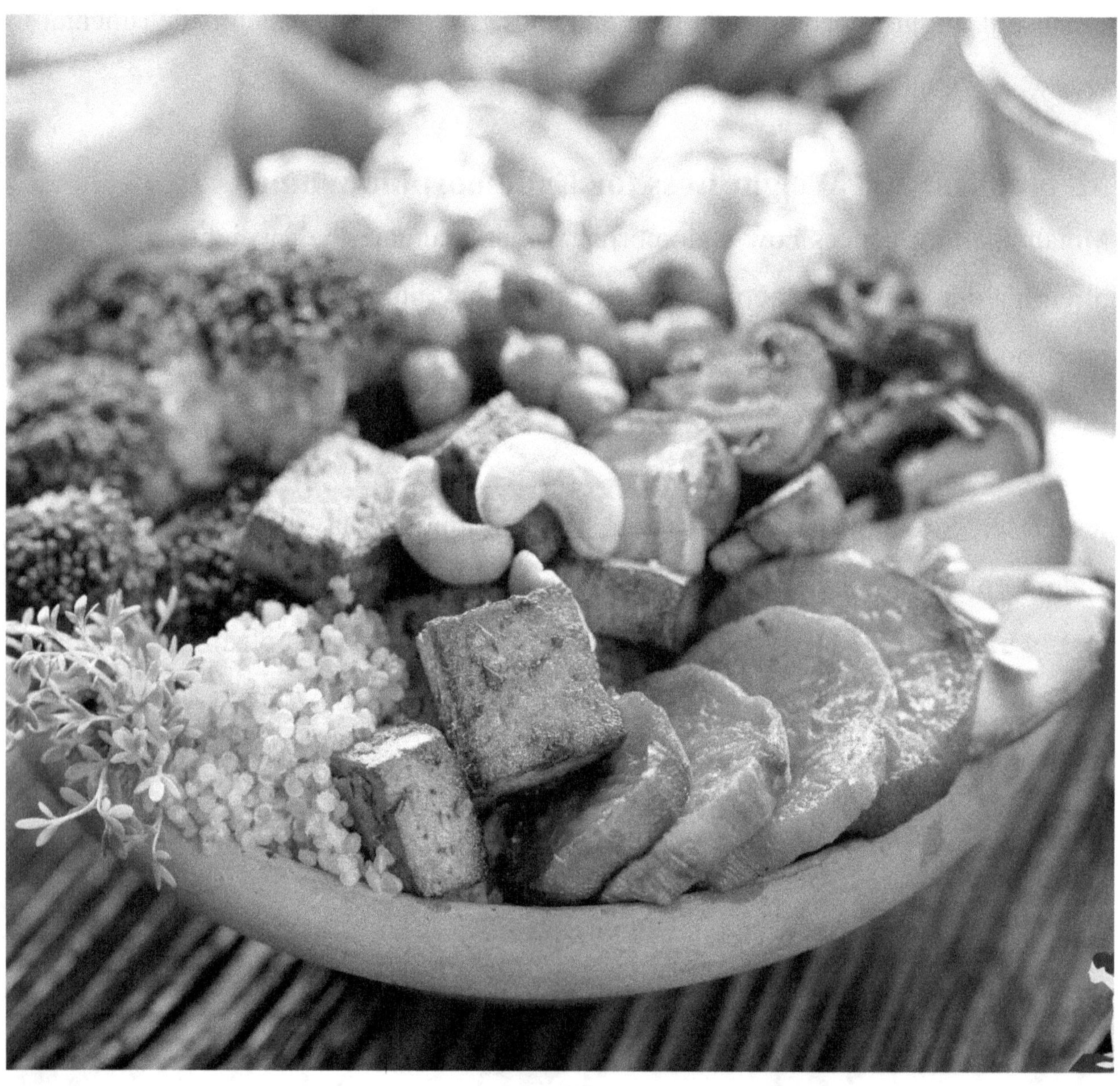

PART 1: THE METABOLIC CONFUSION PLAN

How Metabolic Confusion Works

The Metabolic Confusion Diet, frequently referred to as a dynamic approach to weight management, is based on the idea of keeping your metabolism "on its toes." By regularly altering your caloric and macro nutrient intake, your body is less likely to adapt, so avoiding the dreaded weight loss plateau. The diet is especially good for endomorph women, who may find it more difficult to lose weight due to their inherent predisposition to accumulate fat. Let's look at how each component of this diet helps you lose weight more effectively and sustainably.

Cycling Between High and Low Calorie Days

The Metabolic Confusion Diet focuses on alternating between high and low-calorie days. This cycling technique keeps your metabolism from becoming acclimated to a regular calorie intake, which can often result in a reduction in metabolic rate. By altering your caloric intake, you essentially "confuse" your body, causing it to continually adapt, potentially resulting in more consistent fat loss.

On high-calorie days, you're urged to eat more to provide your body with the energy it requires, especially if you're doing strenuous physical activity. These days, instead of indulging in junk food, choose nutrient-dense foods that give your body with important vitamins and minerals. High-calorie days can also help you retain muscle mass, which is essential for keeping your metabolism running.

In contrast, low-calorie days cause a caloric deficit, causing your body to burn stored fat for energy. The trick here is moderation—low-calorie days should not leave you feeling starved or overly hungry, but they should be sufficient to trigger your body's fat-burning response. The Metabolic Confusion Diet's effectiveness stems from the balance of high and low-calorie days, which keeps your metabolism active and your energy levels steady.

Carb Cycling: High-Carb and Low-Carb Days

Carb cycling is another key component of the Metabolic Confusion Diet. You change your carbohydrate consumption in the same way as you alternate your calorie intake. This strategy entails alternating between high-carb and low-carb days, allowing your body to benefit from carbs' energy and muscle-preserving properties while avoiding fat storage.

On high-carb days, your body gets a large glycogen boost, which is especially useful if you're doing weight training or other high-intensity workouts. These days give your muscles the nourishment they require to grow and recuperate, which is essential for maintaining lean body mass.

In contrast, low-carb days require your body to rely more on fat for energy. By limiting carbohydrate intake, your insulin levels fall, which can aid in fat loss. However, it is critical not to restrict carbs too severely, as they are still required for overall health and energy levels. The balance of high and low-carb days promotes fat reduction while preserving muscle mass, resulting in a leaner body over time.

Protein Intake: Balanced Muscle Growth and Fat Loss

Protein is essential in the Metabolic Confusion Diet, especially for endomorph women who want to maintain muscle mass while shedding fat. A higher protein consumption promotes muscle growth and repair, which is critical when cycling between different amounts of calorie and carb intake.

Protein should be a consistent part of your diet on both high and low calorie days. It keeps you full, regulates blood sugar levels, and delivers muscle-building nutrients. Muscle tissue burns more calories at rest than fat tissue, thus maintaining muscle mass ensures that your metabolism remains active.

Aim for a well-balanced diet rich in lean meats like chicken, fish, turkey, and eggs, as well as plant-based alternatives like beans and lentils. The issue is to get enough protein to support muscle maintenance without going overboard, which can contribute to weight gain if not managed correctly within your overall calorie objectives.

The Function of Fats in Metabolic Confusion

Fats are sometimes misinterpreted in the context of dieting, although they are an important component of the Metabolic Confusion Diet. Avocados, nuts, seeds, and olive oil include healthy fats, which are essential for hormone production, including hormones that regulate metabolism and hunger.

The Metabolic Confusion Diet makes strategic use of fats. On low-carb days, lipids become a more major source of energy, making up for the lower carbohydrate intake. This adjustment not only improves metabolic health, but it also keeps you full and energised throughout the day.

Focus on healthy, unsaturated fats while keeping portion quantities in check. Fats are high in calories, thus even healthy fats should be ingested sparingly to prevent exceeding your caloric requirements.

Creating Your Personalised Meal Plan

Creating a personalised meal plan is essential for success on the Metabolic Confusion Diet. This strategy should be tailored to your exact caloric needs, exercise level, and personal tastes to ensure long-term sustainability.

Begin by calculating the number of high and low-calorie days you'll have each week. A popular strategy is to have two high-calorie days and five low-calorie days, although this can be modified depending on your success and how your body responds. Once you've established this, base your food plans on these calorie limits.

Your meal plan should include a wide range of nutrient-dense meals, with a focus on lean proteins, healthy fats, and complex carbohydrates. Include plenty of veggies and fruits to obtain enough fibre, vitamins, and minerals. Variety is essential for keeping the diet pleasurable and avoiding vitamin deficits.

Calculate Your Caloric Needs

To construct an effective meal plan, first determine your caloric requirements. This includes calculating your Basal Metabolic Rate (BMR), which is the quantity of calories your body need to function at rest. To calculate your BMR, use the following formula:

For Women:

BMR = 655 + 9.6 × weight in kg + 1.8 × height in cm - 4.7 × age in years.

Once you've calculated your BMR, multiply it by an activity factor to get your Total Daily Energy Expenditure. This offers you an indication of the number of calories required to maintain your present weight.

- Sedentary (little or no exercise): BMR x 1.2.
- Lightly active (1-3 days of exercise/sports per week): BMR × 1.375.
- Moderate activity (3-5 days of moderate exercise/sports per week): BMR multiplied by 1.55.
- BMR multiplied by 1.725 for individuals who engage in intense physical activity 6-7 days per week.
- BMR multiplied by 1.9 for very active individuals, such as those who engage in strenuous exercise, physical jobs, or training twice day.

To reduce weight, you must create a calorie deficit. On low-calorie days, aim for a 20-25% drop in your TDEE. On high-calorie days, eat at or slightly below your TDEE to help with muscle maintenance and energy levels.

Weekly Meal Plan for Beginners

Day	Breakfast	Lunch	Dinner	Snacks
Day 1	Greek Yogurt with Berries & Honey	Grilled Chicken Salad with Olive Oil Dressing	Baked Salmon with Quinoa and Steamed Broccoli	Apple Slices with Almond Butter
Day 2	Oatmeal with Chia Seeds and Blueberries	Turkey and Avocado Wrap	Stir-Fried Tofu with Vegetables	Carrot Sticks with Hummus
Day 3	Veggie Omelette with Whole Grain Toast	Quinoa and Black Bean Salad	Grilled Shrimp with Brown Rice and Asparagus	Greek Yogurt with Honey
Day 4	Smoothie: Spinach, Banana, Protein Powder	Chicken and Quinoa Bowl with Mixed Veggies	Baked Cod with Sweet Potato and Green Beans	Mixed Nuts
Day 5	Scrambled Eggs with Avocado and Salsa	Lentil Soup with Whole Grain Bread	Grilled Steak with Roasted Veggies	Cottage Cheese with Pineapple
Day 6	Whole Grain Waffles with Peanut Butter and Banana	Tuna Salad with Spinach and Olive Oil Dressing	Baked Chicken Thighs with Brown Rice and Broccoli	Mixed Berries with Greek Yogurt
Day 7	Smoothie: Mixed Berries, Spinach, Almond Milk	Turkey and Veggie Wrap	Grilled Salmon with Quinoa and Roasted Veggies	Almonds and Dark Chocolate
Day	Greek Yogurt with	Grilled Chicken	Stir-Fried Beef	Sliced Apple

8	Granola and Strawberries	Caesar Salad	with Brown Rice and Veggies	with Almond Butter
Day 9	Veggie Omelette with Avocado	Chickpea Salad with Feta and Olive Oil	Grilled Shrimp with Zoodles (Zucchini Noodles)	Hummus with Carrot and Celery Sticks
Day 10	Oatmeal with Almonds and Berries	Turkey and Cheese Wrap with Veggies	Baked Salmon with Sweet Potato and Spinach	Mixed Nuts
Day 11	Smoothie: Kale, Mango, Protein Powder	Lentil and Veggie Soup	Grilled Chicken with Quinoa and Steamed Broccoli	Greek Yogurt with Honey
Day 12	Scrambled Eggs with Spinach and Whole Grain Toast	Grilled Steak Salad with Balsamic Vinaigrette	Baked Cod with Quinoa and Green Beans	Cottage Cheese with Pineapple
Day 13	Whole Grain Pancakes with Peanut Butter and Banana	Tuna Salad with Spinach and Olive Oil Dressing	Stir-Fried Tofu with Brown Rice and Veggies	Almonds and Dark Chocolate
Day 14	Smoothie: Mixed Berries, Protein Powder, Almond Milk	Grilled Chicken Wrap with Veggies	Grilled Salmon with Roasted Asparagus and Quinoa	Carrot Sticks with Hummus
Day 15	Greek Yogurt with Nuts and Honey	Quinoa and Black Bean Bowl	Baked Chicken Thighs with Brown Rice and	Sliced Apple with Peanut Butter

	Breakfast	Lunch	Dinner	Snack
			Veggies	
Day 16	Veggie Omelette with Avocado and Salsa	Chickpea and Feta Salad	Grilled Shrimp with Zoodles and Roasted Veggies	Greek Yogurt with Honey
Day 17	Oatmeal with Chia Seeds and Fresh Berries	Turkey and Cheese Wrap	Baked Cod with Sweet Potato and Green Beans	Mixed Nuts
Day 18	Smoothie: Spinach, Banana, Almond Milk	Grilled Chicken Salad with Olive Oil Dressing	Grilled Steak with Roasted Veggies	Cottage Cheese with Pineapple
Day 19	Scrambled Eggs with Avocado and Whole Grain Toast	Lentil and Veggie Soup	Stir-Fried Tofu with Brown Rice and Veggies	Apple Slices with Almond Butter
Day 20	Whole Grain Waffles with Berries and Greek Yogurt	Tuna Salad with Spinach and Olive Oil Dressing	Baked Salmon with Quinoa and Roasted Veggies	Mixed Berries with Greek Yogurt
Day 21	Smoothie: Mixed Berries, Kale, Protein Powder	Grilled Chicken Wrap with Veggies	Baked Chicken Thighs with Brown Rice and Steamed Broccoli	Almonds and Dark Chocolate
Day 22	Greek Yogurt with Granola and Berries	Quinoa and Black Bean Salad	Grilled Shrimp with Zoodles and Roasted Veggies	Hummus with Carrot and Celery Sticks
Day 23	Veggie Omelette with Avocado	Turkey and Cheese Wrap	Baked Cod with Sweet Potato and Green Beans	Cottage Cheese with Pineapple

DAY 24	Oatmeal with Almonds and Fresh Berries	Chickpea Salad with Feta and Olive Oil	Grilled Chicken with Quinoa and Steamed Broccoli	Mixed Nuts
DAY 25	Smoothie: Spinach, Banana, Protein Powder	Grilled Steak Salad with Balsamic Vinaigrette	Stir-Fried Tofu with Brown Rice and Veggies	Greek Yogurt with Honey
DAY 26	Scrambled Eggs with Spinach and Whole Grain Toast	Tuna Salad with Spinach and Olive Oil Dressing	Baked Salmon with Quinoa and Roasted Asparagus	Sliced Apple with Almond Butter
DAY 27	Whole Grain Pancakes with Peanut Butter and Banana	Lentil and Veggie Soup	Grilled Chicken with Quinoa and Steamed Broccoli	Carrot Sticks with Hummus
DAY 28	Smoothie: Mixed Berries, Almond Milk, Protein Powder	Turkey and Veggie Wrap	Grilled Shrimp with Zoodles and Roasted Veggies	Almonds and Dark Chocolate

This plan offers a mix of lower and higher calorie days, aligning with the metabolic confusion approach. Adjust portion sizes if necessary to meet specific caloric needs or preferences.

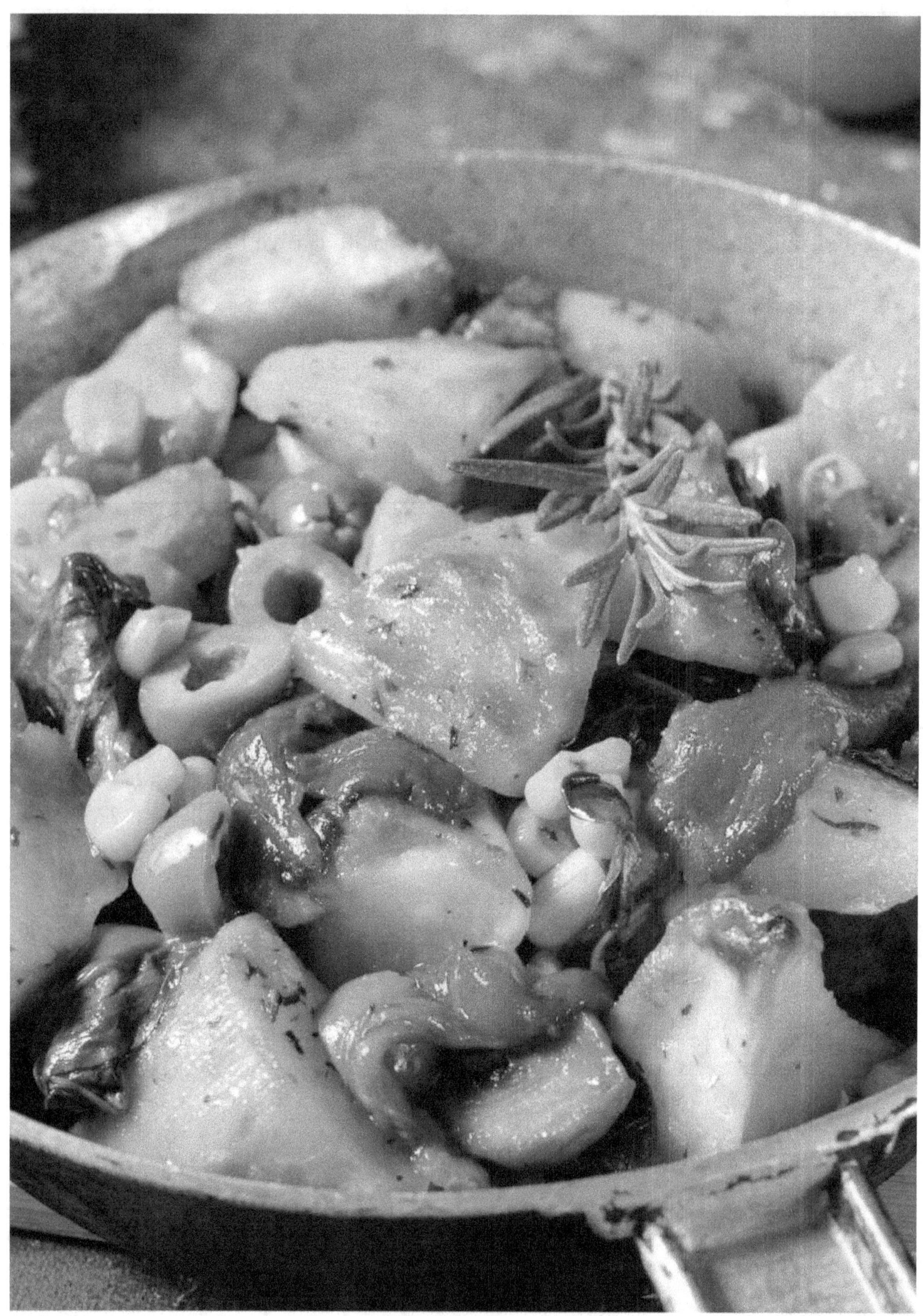

PART 2: BREAKFAST RECIPES

High-Calorie Breakfasts

Avocado and Egg Breakfast Bowl

Ingredients:

1 ripe avocado

2 large eggs

1 tablespoon olive oil

1/4 cup cherry tomatoes, halved

1/4 cup spinach leaves

1 tablespoon fresh chives, chopped (optional)

Salt and pepper to taste

Prep Time:10 minutes

Calories per Serving: 350 calories

Nutritional Information (per serving):

Protein: 15g

Carbohydrates: 14g

Fat: 25g

Fiber: 8g

Sugar: 2g

Instructions:

1. Preparation Ingredients: Cut the avocado in half and remove the pit. Scoop out the flesh and cut or crush it lightly. Wash and halve the cherry tomatoes, then rinse the spinach. To cook eggs, heat olive oil in a nonstick skillet over medium heat. Crack the eggs into a skillet.

2. Cook to your preferred doneness: sunny side up, scrambled, or poached. Season with salt and pepper.

3. Assemble Bowl: Place the avocado slices or mash into a bowl. Garnish with cooked eggs, cherry tomatoes, and spinach leaves.

4. Garnish with chopped chives, if using. Season with more salt and pepper to taste.

5. Serve immediately for a delicious and nutritious breakfast.

Peanut Butter Banana Oatmeal

Ingredients:

1 cup rolled oats

2 cups unsweetened almond milk (or any milk of choice)

1 ripe banana, sliced

2 tbsp natural peanut butter

1 tbsp honey or maple syrup (optional)

1/2 tsp ground cinnamon

A pinch of salt

Prep Time: 5 minutes

Cook Time: 10 minutes

Total Time: 15 minutes

Calories per Serving: 350 calories

Nutritional Information (per serving):

Protein: 10g

Carbohydrates: 50g

Fat: 12g

Fiber: 7g

Sugar: 14g

Instructions:

1. Bring almond milk to a boil in a medium saucepan over medium heat.

2. Stir in the oats and lower the heat to a simmer. Cook for 5–7 minutes, stirring occasionally, until the oats are soft.

3. Combine the sliced bananas, peanut butter, cinnamon, and salt.

4. Stir until the peanut butter is completely blended and the banana is slightly softened. If desired, sweeten with honey or maple syrup. Remove from heat and let aside for a minute before serving.

Greek Yogurt Parfait with Nuts and Berries

Ingredients:

1 cup plain Greek yogurt

1/2 cup fresh mixed berries (blueberries, raspberries, strawberries)

1/4 cup mixed nuts (almonds, walnuts, pecans), chopped

1 tablespoon honey or maple syrup (optional)

1 tablespoon chia seeds (optional for extra nutrition)

Prep Time: 5 minutes

Calories per Serving: 250 calories

Nutritional Information (per serving):

Protein: 14g

Fat: 15g

Carbohydrates: 18g

Fiber: 4g

Sugar: 12g (natural sugars from yogurt and fruit)

Instructions:

1. Layer Yoghurt: Place Greek yoghurt in a glass or bowl.

2. Add Berries: Garnish with fresh mixed berries. Sprinkle Nuts: Spread chopped nuts over the berries.

3. Drizzle Sweetener: If using, add honey or maple syrup. Sprinkle chia seeds on top for extra crunch and nutrition.

4. Serve immediately or refrigerate for a fast snack later.

Chia Seed Pudding with Almonds and Honey

Ingredients:

1/4 cup chia seeds

1 cup unsweetened almond milk

2 tablespoons honey

1/4 teaspoon vanilla extract

2 tablespoons sliced almonds

Fresh berries (optional, for topping)

Prep Time: 10 minutes

Chill Time: 4 hours or overnight

Calories per Serving: 250

Nutritional Information (per serving):

Protein: 7g

Carbohydrates: 30g

Fat: 12g

Fiber: 10g

Sugar: 16g

Instructions:

1. Mix In a mixing dish, add chia seeds, almond milk, honey, and vanilla essence. Stir thoroughly. Allow the mixture to sit for 5 minutes before stirring again to avoid clumping.

2. Cover the bowl and refrigerate for at least 4 hours or overnight to allow the chia seeds to absorb and thicken.

3. Before serving, mix the custard. Optional toppings include chopped almonds and fresh berries.

4. Enjoy: Scoop into bowls and enjoy!

Sweet Potato and Black Bean Breakfast Hash

Ingredients:

2 medium sweet potatoes, peeled and diced

1 cup black beans (canned or cooked), drained and rinsed

1 red bell pepper, diced

1 small onion, diced

2 cloves garlic, minced

1 tablespoon olive oil

1 teaspoon ground cumin

1/2 teaspoon paprika

1/2 teaspoon chili powder

Salt and pepper to taste

Fresh cilantro, chopped (for garnish)

2 large eggs (optional)

Prep Time: 10 minutes

Cook Time: 20 minutes

Total Time: 30 minutes

Servings: 4

Calories per Serving: 250

Nutritional Information (per serving):

Calories: 250

Protein: 8g

Carbohydrates: 35g

Fiber: 8g

Fat: 8g

Sodium: 350mg

Instructions:

1. In a large skillet, heat the olive oil over medium heat.

2. Cook Sweet Potatoes: Add the diced sweet potatoes. Cook, stirring occasionally, until tender (10-12 minutes).

3. Add Vegetables: Combine onion, bell pepper, and garlic. Cook until the onions are transparent (approximately 5 minutes). Season with cumin, paprika, chilli powder, salt, and pepper. Stir thoroughly.

4. Add beans: Fold in the black beans and simmer until cooked through (approximately 3-4 minutes).

5. Optional Eggs: To increase protein content, create two wells in the hash and crack an egg into each. Cover and heat until the eggs are done to your taste. Garnish with fresh cilantro before serving.

Smoked Salmon and Cream Cheese Bagel

Ingredients

1 whole-grain bagel

2 tablespoons cream cheese

2 ounces smoked salmon

1 tablespoon capers

1/4 red onion, thinly sliced

1/4 avocado, sliced

1 teaspoon lemon juice

Fresh dill, for garnish (optional)

Prep Time: 10 minutes

Calories per Serving: 350 calories

Nutritional Information (per serving)

Protein: 18g

Carbohydrates: 32g

Fat: 18g

Fiber: 6g

Sugar: 4g

Sodium: 1000mg

Instructions

1. Toast Bagel: Cut the bagel in half and toast to your desired amount of crispness. Spread Cream Cheese: Evenly distribute 2 tablespoons cream cheese over the sliced sides of the toasted bagel.

2. Add Salmon: Spread 2 ounces of smoked salmon on top of the cream cheese.

3. Top with toppings: Top the salmon with 1 tablespoon capers, 1/4 thinly sliced red onion, and 1/4 avocado slices. Squeeze 1 teaspoon of lemon juice over the top for extra flavour. Garnish with fresh dill, if preferred. Serve immediately for the freshest flavour.

High-Calorie Protein Smoothie

Ingredients:

1 cup full-fat Greek yogurt

1 cup almond milk (or your preferred milk)

1 scoop vanilla protein powder

1 banana

2 tablespoons natural peanut butter

1 tablespoon chia seeds

1 tablespoon honey or maple syrup (optional for extra sweetness)

1/2 cup frozen berries (blueberries, strawberries, or raspberries)

Ice cubes (optional)

Prep Time: 5 minutes

Calories per Serving: 500-550 kcal

Nutritional Information (per serving):

Protein: 30g

Carbohydrates: 60g

Fats: 20g

Fiber: 10g

Sugar: 25g (includes natural sugars from fruit)

Instructions:

1. Blend Blend together Greek yoghurt, almond milk, protein powder, banana, peanut butter, chia seeds, and frozen berries.

2. Sweeten (optional): If you want your smoothie to be sweeter, add honey or maple syrup. Blend Blend until smooth and creamy. If you prefer a thicker consistency, add some ice cubes. Pour into a glass and drink immediately.

Almond Butter and Banana Toast

Ingredients:

2 slices whole-grain bread

2 tablespoons almond butter

1 medium banana

1 tablespoon chia seeds (optional)

1 teaspoon honey (optional)

Prep Time: 5 minutes

Calories per Serving: 290 calories

Nutritional Information (per serving):

Protein: 8g

Fat: 16g

Carbohydrates: 32g

Fiber: 5g

Sugar: 12g

Instructions:

1. Toast the whole-grain bread pieces to your preferred crispness.

2. Spread Almond Butter: While the toast is still warm, spread 1 tablespoon almond butter over each piece.

3. Slice Banana: Peel and cut the banana into thin circles.

4. Top Toast: Spread the banana slices evenly over the almond butter. Optional toppings include chia seeds and honey. Serve and enjoy immediately!

Quinoa Pancakes with Berries

Ingredients:

1 cup quinoa flakes

1 cup almond milk (or any milk of choice)

2 large eggs

2 tbsp honey or maple syrup

1 tsp vanilla extract

1 tsp baking powder

1/2 tsp salt

1 cup mixed berries (fresh or frozen)

1 tbsp coconut oil (for cooking)

Prep Time: 10 minutes

Cook Time: 15 minutes

Total Time: 25 minutes

Calories per Serving: 250

Nutritional Information (per serving):

Protein: 8g

Fat: 10g

Carbohydrates: 35g

Fiber: 5g

Sugar: 10g

Instructions:

1. In a bowl, combine the quinoa flakes, baking powder, salt, and eggs. Mix in the almond milk, honey, and vanilla essence until smooth. Prepare the pan: Heat a nonstick skillet over medium heat and add the coconut oil.

2. Cook Pancakes: Pour 1/4 cup batter per pancake into a skillet. Cook until bubbles appear on the surface (approximately 2-3 minutes), then turn

and cook for an additional 2 minutes until golden brown.

3. Add Berries: Garnish each pancake with a handful of mixed berries. Serve warm and drizzle with honey or maple syrup, if desired.

Spinach and Feta Omelette

Ingredients:

2 large eggs

1 cup fresh spinach, chopped

¼ cup feta cheese, crumbled

1 small onion, finely chopped

1 clove garlic, minced

1 tbsp olive oil

Salt and pepper, to taste

Prep Time: 10 minutes

Calories per Serving: 290 calories

Nutritional Information (per serving):

Protein: 16g

Fat: 22g

Carbohydrates: 6g

Fiber: 2g

Sugar: 2g

Instructions:

1. Heat Oil: Heat olive oil in a nonstick pan over medium heat.

2. Sauté Veggies: Cook onion and garlic until tender, about 3 minutes. Stir in the spinach and simmer for 2 minutes, or until wilted. Prepare the eggs by beating them in a bowl and seasoning with salt and pepper.

3. Cook Eggs: Pour eggs over the vegetables in the pan. Allow to cook for 2 minutes without stirring.

4. Add feta: Sprinkle feta cheese on one half of the omelette.

5. Fold and Cook: Fold the omelette in half and cook for another 2 minutes, or until the eggs are completely set.

6. Serve: Slide the omelette onto a platter and enjoy!

Cottage Cheese and Fruit Bowl

Ingredients:

1 cup cottage cheese (low-fat)

1/2 cup fresh berries (strawberries, blueberries, or raspberries)

1 small apple, diced

1 tablespoon chia seeds

1 teaspoon honey or agave syrup (optional)

1/4 cup walnuts or almonds, chopped (optional)

Prep Time: 10 minutes

Calories per Serving: 250 kcal

Nutritional Information (per serving):

Protein: 20g

Carbohydrates: 30g

Fat: 8g

Fiber: 6g

Sugars: 15g

Instructions:

1. Prepare the ingredients: Wash the berries and dice the apple. In a bowl, combine the cottage cheese.

2. Top with berries and diced apples. Sprinkle chia seeds and chopped nuts, if desired.

3. Drizzle with honey or agave syrup for extra sweetness.

4. Mix and Serve: Gently combine the ingredients and enjoy!

Sausage and Egg Breakfast Burrito

Ingredients:

2 large eggs

1/2 cup cooked sausage crumbles (choose a low-fat variety)

1/4 cup shredded cheddar cheese

1 small bell pepper, diced

1/4 cup onion, diced

1 tablespoon olive oil

2 whole wheat tortillas

Salt and pepper, to taste

1 tablespoon fresh parsley, chopped (optional)

Prep Time: 10 minutes

Calories per Serving: 350 calories

Nutritional Information (per serving):

Protein: 20g

Fat: 18g

Carbohydrates: 28g

Fiber: 5g

Sugar: 3g

Instructions:

1. In a medium-size skillet, heat the olive oil. Cook for about 5 minutes, or until the diced onion and bell pepper soften.

2. Stir in the sausage crumbles and simmer for another 2 minutes. In a bowl, whisk together the eggs and season with salt and pepper. Pour eggs into a skillet and heat, stirring gently, for about 3 minutes, until scrambled and well cooked.

3. Sprinkle cheese over the egg mixture and allow to melt slightly.

4. Warm the tortillas in a separate pan or microwave for a few seconds. Spoon the egg mixture into the centre of each tortilla.

5. Fold the tortilla's sides over the filling, then roll up from the bottom to form a burrito.

6. Serve warm and garnish with fresh parsley, if preferred.

Blueberry Almond Overnight Oats

Ingredients:

1 cup rolled oats

1 cup unsweetened almond milk

1/2 cup plain Greek yogurt

1/2 cup fresh blueberries

1/4 cup sliced almonds

1 tablespoon chia seeds

1 tablespoon honey or maple syrup

1/2 teaspoon vanilla extract

Prep Time: 10 minutes

Calories per Serving: 280 calories

Nutritional Information (per serving):

Protein: 12g

Carbohydrates: 34g

Fat: 12g

Fiber: 7g

Sugar: 13g

Instructions:

1. In a jar or airtight container, combine the oats, chia seeds, and vanilla extract.

2. Add Liquids: Combine the almond milk and Greek yoghurt. Stir until thoroughly blended. Sweeten with honey or maple syrup. Stir again to combine. Gently fold in the blueberries. Refrigerate: Cover and chill overnight (or for at least 6 hours) to allow the oats to absorb the liquid.

3. Serve: Before eating in the morning, sprinkle with sliced almonds.

Savory Quinoa and Egg Muffins

Ingredients:

1 cup cooked quinoa

6 large eggs

1/2 cup diced bell peppers (any color)

1/2 cup chopped spinach

1/4 cup diced onions

1/4 cup shredded cheese (cheddar or feta)

1 tablespoon olive oil

1/2 teaspoon garlic powder

1/2 teaspoon dried oregano

Salt and pepper to taste

Prep Time: 10 minutes

Cook Time: 20 minutes

Total Time: 30 minutes

Calories per Serving: 150 calories

Nutritional Information:

Protein: 10g

Carbohydrates: 10g

Fat: 8g

Fiber: 2g

Instructions:

1. Preheat your oven to 375°F (190°C). Grease a muffin tray or use paper liners.

2. Prepare Quinoa: If quinoa is not already cooked, cook it according to package instructions.

3. Mix Ingredients: In a mixing dish, whisk the eggs. Combine cooked quinoa, bell peppers, spinach, onions, cheese, garlic powder, oregano, salt, and pepper. Mix well.

4. Fill Muffin Tin: Distribute the mixture evenly among the muffin cups. Bake for 20 minutes, or until the muffins are firm and slightly brown on top. Let the muffins cool slightly before removing them from the tin. Serve warm or room temperature.

Full-Fat Greek Yogurt with Honey and Walnuts

Ingredients:

1 cup full-fat Greek yogurt

2 tablespoons honey

1/4 cup walnuts, chopped

Optional: fresh fruit or a sprinkle of cinnamon

Prep Time: 5 minutes

Calories per Serving: 320 calories

Nutritional Information (per serving):

Protein: 12g

Fat: 25g

Carbohydrates: 22g

Fiber: 2g

Sugar: 21g

Instructions:

1. Spoon Yoghurt: Put 1 cup of Greek yoghurt in a bowl. Add Honey: Drizzle 2 tablespoons honey over the yoghurt. Top with walnuts. Add 1/4 cup chopped walnuts on top.

2. Optional: Garnish with fresh fruit or a touch of cinnamon.

3. Serve immediately or refrigerate for later.

PART 3: LUNCH RECIPES

High-Calorie Lunches

Quinoa and Kale Power Bowl

Ingredients:

1 cup quinoa

2 cups water

1 bunch kale, chopped

1 tablespoon olive oil

1 cup cherry tomatoes, halved

1/2 cup shredded carrots

1/4 cup red onion, thinly sliced

1/4 cup feta cheese (optional)

1/4 cup roasted chickpeas (optional)

For the Dressing:

2 tablespoons olive oil

1 tablespoon lemon juice

1 teaspoon Dijon mustard

1 teaspoon honey

Salt and pepper to taste

Prep Time: 20 minutes

Cook Time: 15 minutes

Total Time: 35 minutes

Calories per Serving: 350

Nutritional Information (per serving):

Protein: 10g

Carbohydrates: 45g

Fat: 14g

Fiber: 7g

Sugars: 6g

Instructions:

1. Cook Quinoa: Rinse 1 cup of quinoa in cool water. In a saucepan, bring 2 cups water to a boil. Add the quinoa, reduce the heat to low, cover, and cook for 15 minutes. Fluff with a fork and set aside to cool.

2. Prepare the kale: While the quinoa is cooking, heat 1 tablespoon olive oil in a pan over medium heat. Add the chopped kale and sauté for 3-4 minutes, or until wilted. Set aside. Make dressing: In a small mixing bowl, combine 2 tablespoons olive oil, 1 tablespoon lemon juice, 1 teaspoon Dijon mustard, 1 teaspoon honey, salt, and pepper.

3. Prepare Bowl: In a large mixing bowl, add cooked quinoa, sautéed kale, cherry tomatoes, shredded carrots, and red onion. Optional toppings include feta cheese and roasted chickpeas. Drizzle dressing over bowl and gently toss to mix. Serve immediately or keep refrigerated for up to three days.

Grilled Chicken and Sweet Potato Salad

Ingredients:

2 large chicken breasts

2 medium sweet potatoes, peeled and cubed

1 tablespoon olive oil

1 teaspoon smoked paprika

1/2 teaspoon garlic powder

1/2 teaspoon onion powder

Salt and pepper to taste

4 cups mixed greens (e.g., spinach, arugula, lettuce)

1/4 cup crumbled feta cheese

1/4 cup chopped walnuts

1/2 red onion, thinly sliced

1/2 cup cherry tomatoes, halved

2 tablespoons balsamic vinaigrette

Prep Time: 15 minutes

Cook Time: 20 minutes

Total Time: 35 minutes

Calories per Serving: 350

Nutritional Information (per serving):

Protein: 30g

Carbohydrates: 35g

Fat: 12g

Fiber: 6g

Instructions:

1. Preheat your grill to medium-high. Toss sweet potato cubes with olive oil, smoked paprika, garlic powder, onion powder, salt, and pepper. Grill sweet potatoes: Place them on the grill. Cook for 10-15 minutes, turning regularly, or until tender and faintly browned. Remove and set aside. Season the chicken breasts with salt and pepper.

2. Grill Chicken: Cook for 6-8 minutes per side, or until completely done (internal temperature 165°F). Allow it to rest for 5 minutes before slicing.

3. Salad: In a large bowl, combine the greens, cherry tomatoes, red onion,

crumbled feta, and walnuts. Toss in the grilled sweet potatoes.

4. Slice Chicken: Place the grilled chicken on top of the salad. To dress the salad, drizzle with balsamic vinaigrette and gently toss. Serve and enjoy your hearty, nutritious salad!

Zucchini Noodles with Pesto and Shrimp

Ingredients:

For the Zucchini Noodles:

3 medium zucchinis, spiralized

1 tablespoon olive oil

Salt and pepper to taste

For the Pesto:

1 cup fresh basil leaves

1/4 cup pine nuts

1/4 cup grated Parmesan cheese

1/4 cup olive oil

2 cloves garlic

Juice of 1 lemon

Salt and pepper to taste

For the Shrimp:

1 pound large shrimp, peeled and deveined

1 tablespoon olive oil

1 teaspoon paprika

1 teaspoon garlic powder

Salt and pepper to taste

Prep Time: 20 minutes

Cook Time: 10 minutes

Total Time: 30 minutes

Calories per Serving: 320

Nutritional Information (per serving):

Protein: 25g

Fat: 22g

Carbohydrates: 10g

Fiber: 4g

Sugar: 5g

Instructions:

1. Make the pesto: Blend basil, pine nuts, Parmesan, garlic, and lemon juice in a food processor. Pulse until finely chopped. While the processor is running, gradually add olive oil until smooth. Season with salt and pepper.

2. Prepare the prawns: Toss the prawns with olive oil, paprika, garlic powder, salt and pepper. Cook in a skillet over medium-high heat. Cook the prawns for

2-3 minutes per side, until pink and opaque.

3. Cook the zucchini noodles: In a large pan, heat the olive oil over medium heat. Add the zucchini noodles and season with salt and pepper. Sauté for 3-4 minutes, until tender but crisp. Combine and serve. Toss zucchini noodles with pesto sauce until evenly coated. Top with cooked prawns. Serve immediately and enjoy!

Turkey and Avocado Wrap

Ingredients:

1 large whole wheat or low-carb tortilla

4 oz (115g) sliced turkey breast

1/2 ripe avocado, sliced

1/2 cup shredded lettuce

1/4 cup sliced cucumber

1/4 cup sliced red bell pepper

2 tablespoons hummus or Greek yogurt (for spread)

Salt and pepper to taste

Prep Time: 10 minutes

Calories per Serving: 350 calories

Nutritional Information (per serving):

Protein: 24g

Carbohydrates: 30g

Fat: 15g

Fiber: 8g

Sugar: 4g

Instructions:

1. Spread the hummus or Greek yoghurt equally on the tortilla. Add the sliced turkey breast to the spread. Place avocado slices, shredded lettuce, cucumber, and red bell pepper on top of the turkey.

2. Season with a pinch of salt and pepper. Roll the tortilla firmly, folding the sides to retain the filling within. Cut the wrap in half and eat immediately, or pack it for a fast dinner.

Mediterranean Chickpea Salad

Ingredients

1 can (15 oz) chickpeas, drained and rinsed

1 cup cherry tomatoes, halved

1 cucumber, diced

1/4 red onion, finely chopped

1/4 cup Kalamata olives, sliced

1/4 cup feta cheese, crumbled

2 tbsp extra virgin olive oil

1 tbsp lemon juice

1 tsp dried oregano

Salt and pepper, to taste

Prep Time: 15 minutes

Calories per Serving: 220 calories

Nutritional Information (per serving)

Protein: 8g

Carbohydrates: 20g

Fat: 12g

Fiber: 6g

Sugar: 4g

Instructions:

1. In a large mixing basin, combine chickpeas, cherry tomatoes, cucumber, red onion, and olives.

2. Place feta cheese on top. In a small bowl, combine the olive oil, lemon juice, oregano, salt, and pepper.

3. Pour the dressing over the salad and toss to mix. Serve immediately or refrigerate for 30 minutes before serving.

Salmon and Asparagus Foil Packets

Ingredients:

4 salmon fillets (6 oz each)

1 bunch of asparagus, trimmed

1 lemon, sliced

4 cloves garlic, minced

2 tbsp olive oil

1 tsp dried thyme

1 tsp dried rosemary

Salt and pepper to taste

Prep Time: 15 minutes

Cook Time: 20 minutes

Total Time: 35 minutes

Calories per Serving: 300

Nutritional Information (per serving):

Protein: 30g

Fat: 15g

Carbohydrates: 8g

Fiber: 4g

Sugar: 2g

Instructions:

1. Preheat your oven to 400°F (200°C).
2. Prepare Foil: Cut four huge pieces of aluminium foil. Place them flat on your workspace.
3. Season Vegetables: Toss the asparagus with 1 tablespoon olive oil, half the garlic, thyme, rosemary, salt, and pepper. Place an equal amount of asparagus in the centre of each foil piece.
4. Season Salmon: Drizzle the salmon fillets with the remaining olive oil and garlic. Sprinkle with salt, pepper, and extra thyme and rosemary, if desired. Place one lemon slice on top of each fillet. Assemble the packets by placing a salmon fillet on top of the asparagus on each foil piece. Fold the foil over the salmon and asparagus, then seal the edges tightly to make a packet.
5. Cook: Place the foil packets on a baking sheet and bake for 20 minutes, or until the salmon is fully cooked and readily flaked with a fork.
6. Serve: Carefully open the foil packets (look out for steam) and serve the salmon and asparagus straight from the foil or on a dish.

Lentil and Vegetable Soup

Ingredients:

1 cup dried lentils, rinsed

2 tablespoons olive oil

1 medium onion, chopped

2 garlic cloves, minced

2 carrots, diced

2 celery stalks, diced

1 red bell pepper, diced

1 zucchini, diced

1 cup chopped tomatoes (fresh or canned)

6 cups vegetable broth

1 teaspoon dried thyme

1 teaspoon ground cumin

1 bay leaf

Salt and pepper to taste

2 cups spinach or kale (optional)

Prep Time: 15 minutes

Cook Time: 30 minutes

Total Time: 45 minutes

Servings: 6

Calories per Serving: 180

Nutritional Information (per serving):

Protein: 10g

Carbohydrates: 30g

Fat: 4g

Fiber: 10g

Sugar: 6g

Sodium: 600mg (depending on broth used)

Instructions:

1. Sauté: Heat olive oil in a big pot over medium heat. Cook for 5 minutes, or until the onion and garlic are softened.

2. Add vegetables: Stir in the carrots, celery, bell peppers, and zucchini. Cook for another five minutes. Combine the lentils, chopped tomatoes, vegetable broth, thyme, cumin, and bay leaf. Stir thoroughly.

3. Simmer: Bring to a boil, then reduce the heat to low. Simmer for 25-30 minutes, until the lentils and veggies are soft.

4. Season: Remove the bay leaf. Season with salt and pepper to taste.

5. Optional: Add the spinach or kale and simmer for another 5 minutes, or until wilted. Ladle soup into bowls and enjoy while still warm.

Spaghetti Squash with Turkey Bolognese

Ingredients

1 medium spaghetti squash

1 lb (450g) ground turkey

1 onion, finely chopped

2 cloves garlic, minced

1 carrot, finely chopped

1 celery stalk, finely chopped

1 can (14.5 oz) diced tomatoes

2 tbsp tomato paste

1 cup chicken or vegetable broth

1 tsp dried basil

1 tsp dried oregano

Salt and pepper, to taste

2 tbsp olive oil

Prep Time: 15 minutes

Cook Time: 45 minutes

Total Time: 1 hour

Calories per Serving: 300 calories

Nutritional Information (per serving)

Protein: 24g

Carbohydrates: 25g

Fat: 10g

Fiber: 6g

Sugar: 6g

Instructions:

1. Preheat your oven to 400°F (200°C).

2. Prepare Squash: Divide the spaghetti squash in half lengthwise. Scoop out and discard the seeds. Brush the cut sides with olive oil and set them cut side down on a baking pan. Roast for 40 minutes, or until tender.

3. Cook Bolognese Sauce: In a large skillet, heat olive oil over medium heat. Combine the diced onion, garlic, carrot, and celery. Sauté until softened, about 5 minutes. Add the ground turkey. Cook until browned, then break it up with a spoon. Combine the diced tomatoes, tomato paste, broth, basil, oregano, salt, and pepper. Simmer for 15-20 minutes, stirring periodically, until thick. Prepare spaghetti squash: After roasting the squash, use a fork to scrape the strands into a basin.

4. Serve: Top the spaghetti squash with turkey Bolognese sauce. Garnish with fresh herbs if desired.

Eggplant and Chickpea Stew

Ingredients:

1 large eggplant, diced

1 can (15 oz) chickpeas, drained and rinsed

1 large onion, chopped

3 cloves garlic, minced

1 red bell pepper, chopped

1 can (14.5 oz) diced tomatoes

2 tbsp olive oil

1 tsp ground cumin

1 tsp paprika

1/2 tsp ground turmeric

1/2 tsp cayenne pepper (optional for heat)

Salt and pepper to taste

2 cups vegetable broth

1/4 cup fresh parsley, chopped (for garnish)

Prep Time: 15 minutes

Cook Time: 30 minutes

Total Time: 45 minutes

Calories per Serving: 250 calories (serves 4)

Nutritional Information (per serving):

Protein: 8g

Carbohydrates: 30g

Fat: 12g

Fiber: 9g

Sugar: 8g

Instructions:

1. Heat Oil: In a big pot, heat olive oil over medium heat.

2. Sauté Aromatics: Add the chopped onion and garlic. Cook for approximately 5 minutes, or until the onion is transparent.

3. Add vegetables: Stir in the diced eggplant and red pepper. Cook for 5 minutes or until slightly softened. Season with cumin, paprika, turmeric, cayenne pepper (optional), salt, and pepper. Mix well. Add tomatoes and chickpeas. Pour in the diced tomatoes and chickpeas. Stir to mix.

4. Simmer: Pour in the veggie broth and bring to a boil. Reduce heat and simmer for 20 minutes, or until

aubergine is soft. Taste and adjust seasoning as needed.

5. Garnish and Serve: Stir in fresh parsley right before serving.

Chicken Caesar Salad with Greek Yogurt Dressing

Ingredients:

For the Salad:

2 cups romaine lettuce, chopped

1 cup cherry tomatoes, halved

1 cup grilled chicken breast, sliced

1/4 cup Parmesan cheese, shaved

1/4 cup croutons (optional)

For the Greek Yogurt Dressing:

1/2 cup Greek yogurt (plain, non-fat)

2 tbsp lemon juice

1 tbsp Dijon mustard

1 tbsp olive oil

1 garlic clove, minced

1/4 tsp salt

1/4 tsp black pepper

Prep Time: 15 minutes

Calories per Serving: 350

Nutritional Information (per serving):

Protein: 30g

Carbs: 10g

Fat: 20g

Fiber: 4g

Instructions:

1. Prepare the dressing. In a bowl, combine the Greek yoghurt, lemon juice, Dijon mustard, olive oil, garlic, salt, and pepper. Stir until smooth and blended.

2. Prepare the Salad: Place the chopped romaine lettuce in a large salad bowl. Top with cherry tomatoes, grilled chicken, and Parmesan. Drizzle with Greek yoghurt dressing.

3. Add Croutons (optional): If desired, sprinkle croutons over top for added crunch.

4. Toss & Serve: Gently toss the salad to blend the ingredients and drizzle with the dressing. Serve immediately and enjoy!

Tofu Stir-Fry with Broccoli and Peppers

Ingredients:

1 block (14 oz) extra-firm tofu

2 tablespoons soy sauce

1 tablespoon sesame oil

1 tablespoon olive oil

1 red bell pepper, sliced

1 yellow bell pepper, sliced

2 cups broccoli florets

2 cloves garlic, minced

1 teaspoon fresh ginger, minced

2 tablespoons hoisin sauce

1 tablespoon rice vinegar

1 tablespoon sesame seeds (optional)

2 green onions, sliced (optional)

Prep Time: 15 minutes

Cooking Time: 15 minutes

Total Time: 30 minutes

Calories per Serving: 250 calories

Nutritional Information (per serving):

Protein: 15g

Carbohydrates: 20g

Fat: 15g

Fiber: 5g

Sugar: 8g

Instructions:

1. Preparing Tofu: Drain and squeeze the tofu to remove any extra water. Cut into bite-size chunks.

2. Marinate Tofu: In a bowl, combine tofu cubes and 1 tablespoon soy sauce. Let it sit for 5 minutes. To cook tofu, heat 1 tablespoon sesame oil in a skillet over medium heat. Cook the tofu, turning periodically, until brown and crispy, about 8 minutes. Remove from the pan and set aside.

3. Stir-Fry Vegetables: Add olive oil to the same pan. Sauté the garlic and ginger for one minute. Stir in the bell peppers and broccoli, and cook for 5-7 minutes, or until tender and crisp. Combine the ingredients and return the tofu to the pan. Stir in hoisin sauce, rice vinegar, and the remaining 1 tablespoon soy sauce. Cook for an additional 2-3 minutes, until thoroughly cooked and well mixed. Garnish with sesame seeds and green onions as desired. Serve hot.

Grilled Tuna Steak with Mango Salsa

Ingredients:

For the Tuna Steak:

2 tuna steaks (6 oz each)

2 tbsp olive oil

1 tsp garlic powder

1 tsp paprika

Salt and black pepper to taste

Lemon wedges for serving

For the Mango Salsa:

1 ripe mango, peeled and diced

1/2 red bell pepper, finely chopped

1/4 red onion, finely chopped

1 small jalapeño, seeded and minced

2 tbsp fresh cilantro, chopped

Juice of 1 lime

Salt to taste

Prep Time: 20 minutes

Cook Time: 8 minutes

Total Time: 28 minutes

Calories per Serving: 350

Nutritional Information (per serving):

Protein: 30g

Fat: 22g

Carbohydrates: 16g

Fiber: 4g

Sugar: 12g

Instructions:

1. Preheat your grill to medium-high. Prepare tuna steaks by brushing them with olive oil. Season with garlic powder, paprika, salt, and black pepper.

2. Grill Tuna: Place the steaks on the grill. Cook for 3-4 minutes per side for medium-rare, or longer if you prefer. To make salsa, combine mango, bell pepper, red onion, jalapeño, cilantro, lime juice, and salt.

3. Top the grilled tuna with mango salsa. Garnish with lemon wedges. Enjoy!

Baked Cod with Quinoa and Steamed Veggies

Ingredients

For the Cod:

4 cod fillets (about 6 oz each)

1 tablespoon olive oil

1 lemon, sliced

1 teaspoon dried thyme

1 teaspoon dried oregano

Salt and pepper to taste

For the Quinoa:

1 cup quinoa

2 cups water or low-sodium vegetable broth

1 tablespoon olive oil

1/4 teaspoon salt

For the Steamed Veggies:

1 cup broccoli florets

1 cup carrot slices

1 cup bell pepper strips

Total Time: 30 minutes

Prep Time: 10 minutes

Cook Time: 20 minutes

Calories per Serving: 350

Nutritional Information (per serving)

Protein: 30g

Carbohydrates: 30g

Fat: 10g

Fiber: 5g

Instructions

1. Preheat oven to 400°F (200°C).

2. Prepare cod: Place the cod fillets on a baking sheet. Brush with olive oil, then season with thyme, oregano, salt, and pepper. Top with lemon slices. Bake for 15-20 minutes, or until the fish flakes easily.

3. Cook Quinoa: Rinse the quinoa under cool water. In a pot, combine water or broth, olive oil, and salt. Bring to a boil, then reduce the heat and simmer for 15 minutes, or until the liquid has been absorbed. Fluff with a fork. Steam Vegetables: Fill a small pot with water and heat until it boils. Place the vegetables in a steamer basket over boiling water. Steam for 5-7 minutes, until tender.

4. Assembly Plate: Serve cod fillets with quinoa and steamed vegetables.

Beef and Broccoli Stir-Fry

Ingredients:

1 lb (450g) flank steak, thinly sliced

2 cups broccoli florets

1 red bell pepper, sliced

1 cup snap peas

2 tbsp olive oil

3 cloves garlic, minced

1 tbsp fresh ginger, minced

1/4 cup low-sodium soy sauce

2 tbsp oyster sauce (optional)

1 tbsp rice vinegar

1 tsp sesame oil

1 tbsp cornstarch mixed with 2 tbsp water (for thickening)

Salt and pepper to taste

1 tsp sesame seeds (for garnish)

Prep Time:10 minutes

Cook Time:15 minutes

Calories per Serving: 300 calories

Nutritional Information (per serving):

Protein: 25g

Carbohydrates: 15g

Fat: 15g

Fiber: 4g

Instructions:

1. Prepare ingredients by slicing steak, broccoli, bell pepper, and snap peas.

2. Heat Oil: In a big pan or wok, heat olive oil over medium-high heat.

3. Heat Beef: Add steak pieces and heat for 5 minutes, or until browned. Remove from the pan and set aside.

4. Stir-Fry Vegetables: In the same pan, sauté garlic and ginger for 30 seconds. Combine broccoli, bell pepper, and snap peas. Cook for 3-4 minutes, until the vegetables are soft and crisp. Combine ingredients and return beef to the pan. Combine the soy sauce, oyster sauce (if using), rice vinegar, and sesame oil. Stir thoroughly to coat.

5. Thicken Sauce: Add the cornflour mixture to the pan and stir regularly until thickened, about 1-2 minutes. Season and serve with salt and pepper. Garnish with sesame seeds. Serve hot.

Caprese Salad with Grilled Chicken

Ingredients:

2 boneless, skinless chicken breasts

2 tablespoons olive oil

1 teaspoon dried oregano

Salt and pepper to taste

1 large tomato, sliced

1 ball of fresh mozzarella cheese, sliced

1/4 cup fresh basil leaves

1 tablespoon balsamic vinegar

1 tablespoon honey (optional, for a touch of sweetness)

Prep Time: 20 minutes

Cook Time: 10 minutes

Total Time: 30 minutes

Calories per Serving: 350 calories

Nutritional Information (per serving):

Protein: 30g

Fat: 20g

Carbohydrates: 10g

Fiber: 2g

Sugars: 8g

Instructions:

1. Preheat your grill to medium-high.

2. Season chicken: Brush the chicken breasts with olive oil. Season with dried oregano, salt, and pepper. Grill chicken for 5-7 minutes on each side, or until completely cooked and the internal temperature reaches 165°F (74°C). Rest for 5 minutes before slicing.

3. Assemble salad: On a plate, combine tomato slices, mozzarella slices, and fresh basil leaves.

4. Slice Chicken: Cut the grilled chicken into strips and arrange on top of the salad.

5. Add Dressing: Drizzle the salad with balsamic vinegar and (if using) honey.

6. Enjoy immediately, or refrigerate until ready to serve.

PART 4: DINNER RECIPES

High-Calorie Dinners

Creamy Garlic Butter Shrimp Pasta

Ingredients:

8 oz (225g) pasta (spaghetti or fettuccine)

1 lb (450g) large shrimp, peeled and deveined

2 tbsp butter

3 cloves garlic, minced

1/2 cup heavy cream

1/4 cup chicken broth

1/2 cup grated Parmesan cheese

1 tbsp olive oil

1/2 tsp paprika

Salt and pepper to taste

1 tbsp chopped fresh parsley (optional, for garnish)

Prep Time: 15 minutes

Cooking Time: 15 minutes

Total Time: 30 minutes

Calories per Serving: 450 calories

Nutritional Information (per serving):

Protein: 30g

Carbohydrates: 45g

Fat: 20g

Fiber: 2g

Sugar: 3g

Instructions:

1. Cook pasta in a large pot of salted boiling water until al dente, as directed on the package. Drain and set aside. To cook prawns, heat olive oil in a large skillet over medium heat. Add the prawns and cook for 2-3 minutes per side, or until pink and opaque. Remove from the skillet and set aside.

2. Make Garlic Butter Sauce: In the same skillet, melt the butter over medium heat. Add the minced garlic and simmer for 1 minute, until fragrant.

3. Add liquids: Pour in the heavy cream and chicken broth. Stir well and heat to a simmer. Combine the

ingredients: Add the Parmesan cheese to the skillet and whisk until melted and creamy. Season with paprika, salt, and pepper.

4. Mix Pasta and Shrimp: Return the cooked shrimp to the skillet and stir in the sauce. Add the cooked pasta and toss until evenly coated. Garnish with chopped parsley, if preferred. Serve immediately.

Loaded Sweet Potato and Chicken Casserole

Ingredients:

2 large sweet potatoes, peeled and cubed

2 tbsp olive oil

1 lb (450g) chicken breast, diced

1 red bell pepper, chopped

1 cup broccoli florets

1 cup shredded cheddar cheese

1/2 cup Greek yogurt

1 tbsp garlic powder

1 tsp paprika

1/2 tsp ground cumin

Salt and pepper, to taste

Fresh parsley, for garnish

Prep Time: 15 minutes

Cook Time: 35 minutes

Total Time: 50 minutes

Servings: 4

Calories per Serving: 320

Nutritional Information (per serving):

Protein: 28g

Carbohydrates: 27g

Fat: 12g

Fiber: 6g

Sugars: 8g

Instructions:

1. Preheat your oven to 400°F (200°C). Cook Sweet Potatoes: In salted water, boil sweet potato cubes for 10 minutes or until soft. Drain and mash slightly. To sauté chicken, heat olive oil in a skillet over medium heat. Combine the diced chicken, garlic powder, paprika, cumin, salt, and pepper. Cook until the chicken is no longer pink, about 7-8 minutes.

2. Ingredients: In a large bowl, combine cooked chicken, diced bell

pepper, broccoli, and mashed sweet potatoes. Stir in the Greek yoghurt and half of the cheddar cheese.

3. Assemble Casserole: Place the mixture in a baking dish. Top with the remaining cheddar cheese. Bake the dish for 25 minutes, or until the cheese is melted and bubbling. Garnish and serve with fresh parsley. Serve hot.

Beef and Broccoli Stir-Fry with Jasmine Rice

Ingredients:

For the Stir-Fry:

1 lb (450 g) beef sirloin, thinly sliced

2 cups broccoli florets

2 tbsp vegetable oil

3 cloves garlic, minced

1 tbsp fresh ginger, minced

1/4 cup soy sauce (low sodium)

2 tbsp oyster sauce

1 tbsp hoisin sauce

1 tbsp cornstarch mixed with 2 tbsp water (slurry)

Salt and pepper to taste

1/4 tsp red pepper flakes (optional)

For the Jasmine Rice:

1 cup jasmine rice

1 1/2 cups water

Prep Time:

Total: 30 minutes

Calories per Serving: 300

Jasmine Rice: 150 calories per serving

Nutritional Information (per serving):

Beef and Broccoli Stir-Fry:

Protein: 22 g

Carbohydrates: 14 g

Fat: 18 g

Fiber: 3 g

Jasmine Rice:

Protein: 3 g

Carbohydrates: 33 g

Fat: 0 g

Fiber: 1 g

Instructions:

1. Cook the rice: Rinse 1 cup of jasmine rice in cool water. In a pot, combine the rice with 1 1/2 cups of water. Bring to a boil, then cover

and lower the heat to low. Simmer for fifteen minutes. Remove from heat and cover for 5 minutes.

2. Prepare the stir-fry: Heat 2 tablespoons vegetable oil in a large pan or wok over medium-high heat. Cook 1 pound of thinly sliced beef for 3-4 minutes, or until browned. Remove the beef and set aside. In the same pan, combine the minced garlic and ginger. Sauté for thirty seconds. Add 2 cups broccoli florets and simmer for 3 minutes, or until tender-crisp. Return the beef to the pan. Combine 1/4 cup soy sauce, 2 tablespoons oyster sauce, and 1 tablespoon hoisin sauce. Stir to coat. Cook for around 2 minutes, stirring in the cornflour slurry until the sauce thickens. Season with salt, pepper, and red pepper flakes, if desired.

3. Serve: Fluff the jasmine rice with a fork. Serve the stir-fry on a bed of jasmine rice.

Cheesy Baked Ziti with Ground Beef

Ingredients:

12 oz ziti pasta

1 lb ground beef

1 small onion, finely chopped

2 cloves garlic, minced

1 jar (24 oz) marinara sauce

1 can (14.5 oz) diced tomatoes

1 tsp dried basil

1 tsp dried oregano

1/2 tsp salt

1/4 tsp black pepper

1 cup ricotta cheese

1 1/2 cups shredded mozzarella cheese

1/2 cup grated Parmesan cheese

2 tbsp olive oil

Prep Time: 15 minutes

Cook Time: 30 minutes

Total Time: 45 minutes

Servings: 6

Calories per Serving: 400 kcal

Nutritional Information (per serving):

Protein: 22 g

Carbohydrates: 40 g

Fat: 18 g

Fiber: 3 g

Sugars: 8 g

Instructions:

1. Preheat your oven to 375°F (190°C). Cook pasta: Cook ziti in salted water according to package directions. Drain and set aside.

2. Prepare the Beef Mixture: Heat olive oil in a large skillet over medium heat. Combine ground meat, onion, and garlic. Cook until the steak is browned and the onion softens. Drain any extra fat.

3. Add Sauce: Combine marinara sauce, diced tomatoes, basil, oregano, salt, and pepper. Simmer for five minutes.

4. Ingredients: Combine cooked ziti and beef sauce. In a large mixing bowl, combine ricotta cheese and 1 cup mozzarella cheese. In a baking dish, spread a layer of the ziti mixture. Top with the ricotta cheese mixture. Sprinkle the remaining mozzarella and parmesan cheese on top. Bake in the oven for 20-25 minutes, until the cheese is bubbling and golden. Allow the ziti to cool for a few minutes before serving. Enjoy!

Creamy Chicken Alfredo with Spinach

Ingredients:

2 large chicken breasts, sliced

2 tablespoons olive oil

3 cloves garlic, minced

1 cup heavy cream

1 cup grated Parmesan cheese

1/2 cup chicken broth

2 cups fresh spinach

1 teaspoon dried Italian herbs

Salt and pepper to taste

8 oz whole wheat or low-carb fettuccine (optional)

Prep Time: 10 minutes

Cook Time: 20 minutes

Total Time: 30 minutes

Servings: 4

Nutritional Information (per serving):

Calories: 400

Protein: 34g

Fat: 28g

Carbohydrates: 8g

Fiber: 2g

Net Carbs: 6g

Instructions:

1. To cook the chicken, heat olive oil in a large skillet over medium heat. Add the sliced chicken breasts, season with salt & pepper, and cook for 6-7 minutes per side, until golden and cooked through. Remove and set aside.

2. Prepare the sauce: In the same skillet, saute the minced garlic for about 1 minute, until aromatic. Combine heavy cream and chicken broth. Bring to a simmer and stir occasionally.

3. Add Cheese: Gradually mix in the grated Parmesan until the sauce is smooth and creamy. Season with Italian herbs, salt, and pepper as desired.

4. Incorporate Spinach: Cook fresh spinach in a skillet until wilted, about 2 minutes.

5. Combine Chicken and Sauce: Return the cooked chicken to the skillet and coat it with the creamy sauce. Simmer for an additional two minutes.

6. Optional Fettuccine: Cook fettuccine according to package instructions. Toss with the creamy chicken Alfredo sauce and serve on the side.

7. Serving: Spoon the creamy chicken Alfredo with spinach onto plates. If preferred, garnish with additional Parmesan. Enjoy!

Lamb and Potato Shepherd's Pie

Ingredients:

For the Filling:

500g ground lamb

1 medium onion, chopped

2 garlic cloves, minced

2 carrots, diced

1 cup frozen peas

1 cup beef broth

1 tablespoon tomato paste

1 teaspoon dried thyme

1 teaspoon dried rosemary

Salt and pepper to taste

2 tablespoons olive oil

For the Mashed Potato Topping:

4 large potatoes, peeled and cubed

2 tablespoons butter

1/4 cup milk

Salt and pepper to taste

Prep Time: 20 minutes

Cook Time: 45 minutes

Total Time: 1 hour 5 minutes

Calories per Serving: 350 (based on 4 servings)

Nutritional Information per Serving:

Protein: 22g

Carbohydrates: 30g

Fat: 15g

Fiber: 5g

Instructions:

1. Prepare potatoes: Boil potatoes in salted water for 15 minutes, or until tender. Drain and return to the pot. Mash in butter and milk until smooth. Season with salt and pepper. Set aside.

2. Cook Filling: In a large skillet, heat olive oil over medium heat. Combine onions and garlic. Cook until soft. Add ground lamb. Cook until browned, then break it up with a spoon. Stir in the carrots, peas, tomato paste, thyme, rosemary, salt, and pepper. Pour in the beef broth and cook for 10 minutes until thickened.

3. Assemble pie: Preheat the oven to 200°C (400°F). Spoon the lamb mixture into a baking dish. Spread mashed potatoes equally on top.

4. Bake: Bake for 20-25 minutes, or until the top is golden and the filling bubbles.

5. Serve: Let it cool for 5 minutes before serving.

Salmon with Quinoa and Avocado Salad

Ingredients:

For the Salmon:

4 salmon fillets (6 oz each)

2 tbsp olive oil

1 lemon (sliced)

1 tsp dried oregano

Salt and pepper to taste

For the Quinoa Salad:

1 cup quinoa (uncooked)

2 cups water or low-sodium chicken broth

1 ripe avocado (diced)

1 cup cherry tomatoes (halved)

1/4 cup red onion (finely chopped)

1/4 cup fresh parsley (chopped)

2 tbsp olive oil

1 tbsp lemon juice

Salt and pepper to taste

Prep Time: 30 minutes

Calories per Serving: 450

Nutritional Information (per serving):

Protein: 30g

Carbs: 30g

Fats: 25g

Fiber: 8g

Sugars: 4g

Instructions:

1. Preheat your oven to 400°F (200°C).

2. Prepare salmon: Place the salmon fillets on a baking sheet. Drizzle with olive oil, then season with salt, pepper, and dried oregano. Place lemon slices on top of the fillet. Bake for 15-20 minutes, or until the salmon is thoroughly cooked and readily flaked with a fork.

3. Cook Quinoa: Rinse the quinoa under cool water. Heat water or broth in a medium pot until it boils. Add the quinoa, decrease the heat, cover, and cook for 15 minutes. Fluff with a fork and set aside to cool.

4. Prepare salad: In a large mixing dish, combine cooked quinoa, diced avocado, cherry tomatoes, red onion, and parsley. Drizzle with olive oil and lemon juice. Season with salt and pepper, and gently toss to combine.

5. Serve: Place one dish of quinoa salad on each plate. Top with a salmon fillet. If preferred, garnish with more parsley or lemon wedges.

Low-Calorie Dinners

Grilled Lemon Herb Chicken with Steamed Vegetables

Ingredients:

For the Chicken:

4 boneless, skinless chicken breasts

2 tablespoons olive oil

1 lemon, juiced

2 cloves garlic, minced

1 tablespoon dried oregano

1 teaspoon dried thyme

Salt and pepper to taste

For the Vegetables:

1 cup broccoli florets

1 cup carrot slices

1 cup snap peas

1 tablespoon olive oil

Salt and pepper to taste

Prep Time: 15 minutes

Cook Time: 20 minutes

Total Time: 35 minutes

Calories per Serving: 350

Nutritional Information (per serving):

Protein: 30g

Carbohydrates: 20g

Fat: 15g

Fiber: 6g

Sugars: 7g

Instructions:

1. Marinate chicken in a basin with olive oil, lemon juice, minced garlic, oregano, thyme, salt, and pepper. Marinate chicken breasts for at least 15 minutes.

2. Grill Chicken: Heat the grill to medium-high. Grill chicken for 6-7 minutes per side, or until thoroughly done (internal temperature should be

165°F). Allow to rest for a few minutes.

3. Steam Vegetables: While the chicken grills, steam the broccoli, carrots, and snap peas for 5-7 minutes, or until tender-crisp. Drizzle with olive oil, then season with salt and pepper. Slice the grilled chicken and serve with steaming veggies. Enjoy your healthy and delicious lunch!

Zucchini Noodles with Turkey Bolognese

Ingredients:

For the Turkey Bolognese:

1 lb (450g) ground turkey

1 tablespoon olive oil

1 onion, finely chopped

2 garlic cloves, minced

1 red bell pepper, diced

1 carrot, diced

1 cup (240ml) crushed tomatoes

2 tablespoons tomato paste

1 teaspoon dried basil

1 teaspoon dried oregano

Salt and pepper to taste

For the Zucchini Noodles:

4 medium zucchinis

1 tablespoon olive oil

Salt and pepper to taste

Prep Time:

Turkey Bolognese: 10 minutes

Zucchini Noodles: 10 minutes

Total: 20 minutes

Calories per Serving: 300

Nutritional Information (per serving):

Protein: 25g

Carbohydrates: 15g

Fat: 15g

Fiber: 4g

Sugar: 8g

Instructions

1. Turkey Bolognese: In a large skillet, heat olive oil over medium heat. Add the diced onion and simmer for about 3 minutes, until transparent. Stir in the minced garlic and simmer for 1 minute. Add the ground turkey and heat until browned. Combine the red bell pepper, carrot, smashed

tomatoes, tomato paste, basil, and oregano. Simmer for 15 minutes, stirring periodically. Season with salt and pepper.

2. Prepare Zucchini Noodles: Zucchini can be spiralised into noodles or peeled. In a large skillet, heat olive oil over medium heat. Add the zucchini noodles and simmer for 3-4 minutes, until cooked. Season with salt and pepper.

3. Serve: Divide the zucchini noodles among plates. Top with turkey Bolognese. Garnish with more basil if desired.

Baked Cod with Asparagus and Cherry Tomatoes

Ingredients:

4 cod fillets (6 oz each)

1 bunch asparagus, trimmed

1 cup cherry tomatoes, halved

2 tablespoons olive oil

1 lemon, sliced

3 cloves garlic, minced

1 teaspoon dried thyme

1 teaspoon dried basil

Salt and pepper to taste

Prep Time: 10 minutes

Cook Time: 20 minutes

Calories per Serving: 250 calories

Nutritional Information (per serving):

Protein: 32g

Carbohydrates: 10g

Fat: 10g

Fiber: 4g

Instructions:

1. Preheat oven to 400°F (200°C). Prepare vegetables: Spread the asparagus and cherry tomatoes on a baking sheet. Drizzle with 1 tablespoon olive oil, then season with garlic, thyme, basil, salt, and pepper. Toss to coat.

2. Add Cod: Place cod fillets on top of the vegetables. Drizzle with the remaining olive oil, then season with salt and pepper. Place lemon slices over the cod.

3. Roast in the oven for 15-20 minutes, or until the fish is cooked through

and the vegetables are soft. Serve warm.

Quinoa Stuffed Bell Peppers

Ingredients:

4 large bell peppers (any color)

1 cup quinoa

2 cups water or vegetable broth

1 tablespoon olive oil

1 small onion, diced

2 cloves garlic, minced

1 cup corn kernels (fresh or frozen)

1 cup black beans, drained and rinsed

1 cup cherry tomatoes, halved

1 teaspoon ground cumin

1 teaspoon paprika

½ teaspoon chili powder

Salt and pepper to taste

½ cup shredded cheese (optional)

Fresh cilantro for garnish (optional)

Prep Time: 20 minutes

Cook Time: 25 minutes

Total Time: 45 minutes

Calories per Serving: 320

Nutritional Information (per serving, based on 4 servings):

Calories: 320

Protein: 12g

Carbohydrates: 55g

Fat: 7g

Fiber: 8g

Sugar: 7g

Sodium: 300mg

Instructions:

1. Preheat your oven to 375°F (190°C). Cook Quinoa: Rinse the quinoa in cool water. Heat the water or vegetable broth in a medium pot until it boils. Add the quinoa, decrease the heat, cover, and cook for 15 minutes. Fluff with a fork. Prepare the bell peppers by cutting off the tops and removing the seeds. Lightly cover the peppers in olive oil and arrange them upright in a baking tray.

2. Sauté Vegetables: Heat olive oil in a skillet over medium heat. Sauté the onion and garlic until transparent. Combine the corn, black beans,

cherry tomatoes, cumin, paprika, chilli powder, salt and pepper. Cook for five minutes.

3. Mix Filling: Mix cooked quinoa into the sautéed mixture. Stir thoroughly. Stuff the bell peppers with the quinoa mixture. If using cheese, sprinkle it over top. Cover with foil and bake for 20 minutes. Remove the foil and bake for 5 more minutes, or until the peppers are cooked. Garnish and serve: If preferred, add fresh cilantro. Serve warm.

1 tablespoon chopped fresh basil (optional, for garnish)

Prep Time: 15 minutes

Cook Time: 30 minutes

Total Time: 45 minutes

Calories per Serving: 300 calories

Nutritional Information (per serving):

Protein: 22g

Carbohydrates: 25g

Fat: 15g

Fiber: 4g

Sugar: 4g

Spaghetti Squash with Pesto and Grilled Shrimp

Ingredients:

1 medium spaghetti squash

2 tablespoons olive oil

1 cup basil pesto (store-bought or homemade)

1 pound large shrimp, peeled and deveined

1 tablespoon lemon juice

1 teaspoon garlic powder

Salt and pepper to taste

Instructions:

1. Preheat the oven. Preheat your oven to 400°F (200° C). Prepare the spaghetti squash: Cut the squash in half lengthwise, then scrape out the seeds. Brush the inside with 1 tablespoon olive oil and season with salt and pepper. Place the cut side down on a baking sheet and roast for 30 minutes, or until soft.

2. Grill the prawns. While the squash cooks, combine the prawns with

lemon juice, garlic powder, salt and pepper. Heat the remaining 1 tablespoon olive oil in a grill pan over medium-high heat. Grill the prawns for 2-3 minutes per side, until pink and opaque. Prepare the pesto: If you're using store-bought pesto, skip to the following step. To make pesto, combine fresh basil, garlic, pine nuts, Parmesan, and olive oil until smooth.

3. Finish the spaghetti squash: After the squash has cooled enough to handle, use a fork to scrape the flesh into spaghetti-like strands. Combine and serve. Toss the spaghetti squash with pesto until evenly coated. Top with grilled prawns and garnish with fresh basil, if preferred.

Cauliflower Fried Rice with Chicken

Ingredients:

1 medium head of cauliflower, riced

1 cup cooked chicken breast, diced

1 cup mixed vegetables (peas, carrots, corn)

2 cloves garlic, minced

2 green onions, chopped

2 tablespoons soy sauce (low sodium)

1 tablespoon sesame oil

2 large eggs, beaten

Salt and pepper to taste

Prep Time: 15 minutes

Cook Time: 15 minutes

Total Time: 30 minutes

Calories per Serving: 350 calories

Nutritional Information (per serving):

Protein: 30g

Carbohydrates: 20g

Fat: 18g

Fiber: 5g

Sodium: 600mg

<u>Instructions:</u>

1. Prepare the cauliflower: Remove the stalk and pulse the florets in a food processor until rice-sized.

2. Set aside. Cook the chicken in a large pan over medium heat, adding 1 tablespoon sesame oil. Add the diced chicken and heat until browned. Remove and set aside. Sauté the vegetables in the same skillet, adding extra oil as needed. Sauté the minced garlic and chopped green onions until aromatic. Toss in the mixed vegetables and simmer for 3-4 minutes, until tender.

3. Scramble eggs: Move the vegetables to one side of the pan. Pour the beaten eggs into the empty side and scramble until completely done.

4. Combine: Add the riced cauliflower to the pan. Stir well to combine all of the ingredients. Season by pouring soy sauce over the mixture. Stir until evenly coated. Cook for a further 5-7 minutes, until the cauliflower is soft but not mushy.

5. Add Chicken: Return the cooked chicken to the pan. Stir everything together until thoroughly hot. Season with salt and pepper to taste. Garnish with more green onions if preferred and serve hot.

Tofu Stir-Fry with Mixed Vegetables

<u>Ingredients:</u>

1 block firm tofu, drained and cubed

2 tablespoons olive oil

1 red bell pepper, sliced

1 yellow bell pepper, sliced

1 cup broccoli florets

1 cup snap peas

1 medium carrot, thinly sliced

3 cloves garlic, minced

2 tablespoons soy sauce (low sodium)

1 tablespoon hoisin sauce

1 tablespoon rice vinegar

1 teaspoon grated ginger

1 tablespoon sesame seeds (optional)

Cooked brown rice, for serving

Prep Time: 15 minutes

Cook Time: 10 minutes

Total Time: 25 minutes

Calories per Serving: 250

Nutritional Information (per serving):

Protein: 14g

Carbohydrates: 18g

Fat: 15g

Fiber: 4g

Sugar: 6g

Instructions:

1. Prepare the tofu by cutting it into 1-inch pieces. Heat 1 tablespoon olive oil in a large skillet over medium-high heat. Cook the tofu until golden brown on all sides, about 5 minutes. Remove the tofu and leave aside. Stir-Fry Vegetables: In the same skillet, heat the remaining tablespoon of olive oil. Sauté garlic and ginger for 30 seconds. Combine the bell peppers, broccoli, snap peas, and carrot. Stir-fry for about 4-5 minutes, or until the vegetables are soft and crisp.

2. Add sauces: Return the tofu to the skillet. Add in the soy sauce, hoisin sauce, and rice vinegar. Stir thoroughly to coat the tofu and vegetables.

3. Finish and serve: Cook for another 2 minutes, allowing the sauce to thicken slightly. Sprinkle with sesame seeds if preferred. Serve hot with cooked brown rice.

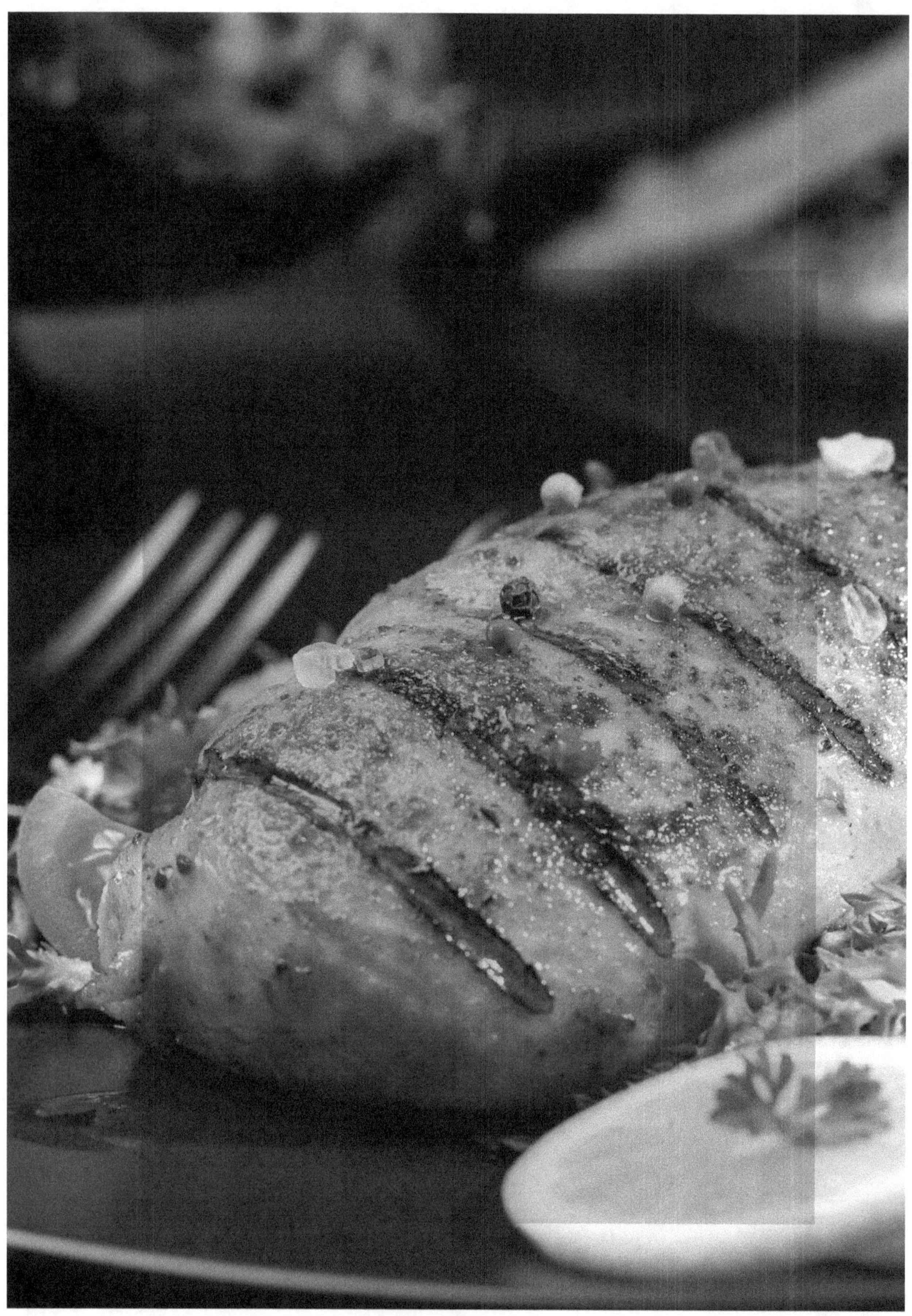

PART 5: SNACKS AND DESSERTS

High-Calorie Snacks and Desserts

Nut Butter and Dark Chocolate Bliss

Ingredients:

1 cup natural almond butter (or peanut butter)

1/2 cup dark chocolate chips (70% cocoa or higher)

2 tablespoons coconut oil

2 tablespoons honey or maple syrup

1/2 teaspoon vanilla extract

Pinch of sea salt

Prep Time: 15 minutes

Chill Time: 30 minutes

Total Time: 45 minutes

Servings: 12 pieces

Calories per Serving: 120 kcal

Nutritional Information (per serving):

Calories: 120 kcal

Protein: 3g

Fat: 10g

Carbohydrates: 6g

Fiber: 2g

Sugar: 4g

Instructions:

1. To melt the ingredients, put dark chocolate chips and coconut oil in a microwave-safe bowl.

2. Microwave in 30-second increments, swirling until completely melted and smooth. Mix in the almond butter, honey, vanilla essence, and a pinch of sea salt until thoroughly incorporated. Fill Moulds: Transfer the mixture to a silicone mould or tiny muffin tin lined with paper liners. Fill each mould approximately halfway.

3. Chill: Refrigerate the mould for about 30 minutes, or until the chocolate is set. Take out the Nut Butter and Dark Chocolate Bliss bits and enjoy!

Greek Yogurt with Honey and Walnuts

Ingredients:

1 cup Greek yogurt (full-fat or low-fat)

2 tablespoons honey

2 tablespoons walnuts, chopped

1/4 teaspoon cinnamon (optional)

Prep Time: 5 minutes

Calories Per Serving: 220 calories

Nutritional Information (per serving):

Protein: 10g

Carbohydrates: 26g

Fat: 10g

Fiber: 1g

Sugars: 23g

Instructions:

1. To prepare, spoon the Greek yoghurt into a bowl.
2. Drizzle the honey on the yoghurt. Sprinkle the chopped walnuts over top. For added flavour, sprinkle with a touch of cinnamon.
3. Stir lightly or consume as is.

Avocado and Tuna Stuffed Baked Potato

Ingredients:

2 large baking potatoes

1 ripe avocado

1 can (5 oz) tuna in water, drained

2 tbsp Greek yogurt (optional)

1 tbsp lemon juice

1 tbsp olive oil

1 small red onion, finely chopped

1 small tomato, diced

Salt and pepper to taste

Fresh parsley, chopped (for garnish)

Prep Time: 10 minutes

Cook Time: 60 minutes

Calories per Serving: 350 kcal

Nutritional Information (per serving):

Protein: 20g

Carbohydrates: 45g

Fat: 15g

Fiber: 8g

Sodium: 300mg

<u>**Instructions:**</u>

1. Preheat the Oven: Preheat to 400°F (200°C). Bake potatoes: Pierce them with a fork. Bake for 60 minutes, or until tender.

2. Prepare the Filling: While the potatoes are baking, mash the avocado in a bowl. Combine tuna, Greek yoghurt, lemon juice, olive oil, red onion, and tomato. Season with salt and pepper.

3. Stuff Potatoes: Once baked, make a slit in the top of each potato. Scoop off part of the insides and combine with the tuna and avocado filling.

4. Fill and serve: Place the mixture back into the potatoes. Garnish with chopped parsley.

5. Enjoy Warm: Serve immediately while the potatoes are still hot.

Homemade Energy Balls

<u>**Ingredients:**</u>

1 cup rolled oats

1/2 cup almond butter

1/4 cup honey

1/4 cup ground flaxseed

1/4 cup dark chocolate chips

1/4 cup chopped almonds

1/4 cup dried cranberries

1/2 tsp vanilla extract

Pinch of salt

Prep Time: 15 minutes

Calories per Serving: 120 calories (1 ball)

Nutritional Information (per serving):

Protein: 3g

Carbohydrates: 12g

Fat: 7g

Fiber: 2g

Sugar: 6g

<u>**Instructions**</u>

1. Combine oats, almond butter, and honey in a large bowl.

2. Combine the flaxseed, chocolate chips, almonds, cranberries, vanilla, and salt. Stir until thoroughly blended.

3. Roll the mixture into little balls approximately an inch in diameter.

4. Chill in the refrigerator for 30 minutes to set. Enjoy as a quick energy boost snack!

Smoothie Bowls with Granola and Nut Butter

Ingredients:

1 cup frozen mixed berries

1 small banana, sliced

1/2 cup unsweetened almond milk

1/4 cup Greek yogurt (optional)

1/4 cup granola

1 tablespoon almond butter (or your favorite nut butter)

1 teaspoon chia seeds (optional)

Fresh berries, banana slices, or coconut flakes for topping

Prep Time: 10 minutes

Calories per Serving: 320 calories

Nutritional Information (per serving):

Protein: 10g

Carbohydrates: 45g

Fiber: 8g

Sugars: 20g

Fat: 12g

Saturated Fat: 2g

Instructions:

1. Blend the frozen berries, banana, almond milk, and Greek yoghurt until smooth.

2. Pour the smoothie into a bowl.

3. Sprinkle with granola, almond butter, and chia seeds.

4. Sprinkle with fresh berries, banana slices, or coconut flakes. Serve immediately. Enjoy!

Cheese and Whole-Grain Crackers

<u>Ingredients:</u>

Whole-Grain Crackers: 8-10 (store-bought or homemade)

Cheese: 2 oz (e.g., sharp cheddar, gouda, or your choice)

Fresh Herbs (optional): A few sprigs of thyme or rosemary

Olive Oil (optional): 1 tsp

Sea Salt (optional): A pinch

Pepper (optional): A pinch

Prep Time: 5 minutes

Calories Per Serving: 150 calories

Nutritional Information (per serving):

Protein: 8 g

Carbohydrates: 15 g

Fat: 8 g

Fiber: 2 g

Calcium: 150 mg

Sodium: 300 mg

<u>Instructions:</u>

1. Prepare the crackers: Place whole grain crackers on a serving tray or platter.

2. Slice the cheese: Cut the cheese into bite-size chunks or thin slices.

3. Assemble: Place a piece of cheese on each cracker. If preferred, drizzle with olive oil, season with sea salt, and add a pinch of pepper. Garnish with fresh herbs to add flavour and elegance.

4. Serve immediately or keep in an airtight jar for up to one day.

Banana with Almond Butter and Dark Chocolate Chips

<u>Ingredients:</u>

1 ripe banana

1 tablespoon almond butter

1 tablespoon dark chocolate chips (70% cocoa or higher)

Prep Time: 5 minutes

Calories per Serving: 200 calories

Nutritional Information (per serving):

Protein: 4 grams

Carbohydrates: 26 grams

Fat: 10 grams

Fiber: 4 grams

Sugar: 14 grams

Instructions:

1. Slice the Banana: Peel and chop the banana into bite-size rounds. Spread a small spoonful of almond butter on each banana slice. Sprinkle Chocolate Chips: Add a few dark chocolate chips to each slice. Serve: Place the pieces on a dish and eat immediately.

Low-Calorie Snacks and Desserts

Greek Yogurt with Berries

Ingredients:

1 cup plain Greek yogurt

1/2 cup mixed berries (strawberries, blueberries, raspberries)

1 tablespoon honey or maple syrup

1 tablespoon chia seeds (optional)

A few fresh mint leaves for garnish (optional)

Prep Time: 5 minutes

Calories per Serving: 150 calories

Nutritional Information (per serving):

Protein: 12g

Carbohydrates: 20g

Fat: 2g

Fiber: 4g

Sugar: 15g

Instructions:

1. Spoon Yoghurt: Place Greek yoghurt in a bowl or serving plate. Top with a combination of berries. Drizzle honey or maple syrup over the fruit and yoghurt.

2. Optional Chia: If using, sprinkle chia seeds. Garnish with mint leaves for a fresh touch if preferred. Serve immediately or refrigerate for later.

Cucumber and Hummus

Ingredients:

1 large cucumber
1 cup hummus (store-bought or homemade)
1 tablespoon chopped fresh dill or parsley (optional)
Salt and pepper to taste

Prep Time: 10 minutes
Calories per Serving: 100 calories per serving

Nutritional Information (per serving):
Fat: 5g
Carbohydrates: 12g
Protein: 3g
Fiber: 3g

Instructions:

1. Wash and cut the cucumber into 1/4-inch-thick circles.
2. Prepare the hummus: If you're using store-bought hummus, whisk it well. If homemade, make sure it's smooth.
3. Assemble: Place cucumber slices on a platter. Top each piece with a dollop or spread of hummus. Garnish with chopped dill or parsley, if desired. Season with a pinch of salt and pepper. Serve immediately or refrigerate for a refreshing, healthful snack.

Apple Slices with Almond Butter

Ingredients:

1 medium apple
2 tablespoons almond butter
1 tablespoon chia seeds (optional)
A sprinkle of cinnamon (optional)

Prep Time: 5 minutes
Calories per Serving: 180

Nutritional Information per Serving:

Calories: 180

Protein: 4g

Carbohydrates: 24g

Fat: 10g

Fiber: 5g

Sugars: 15g

Instructions:

1. Slice the apple: Core and cut the apple into thin, even slices. Spread almond butter on a dish.

2. Dip and enjoy: Dip apple slices in the almond butter.

3. Add extras: If desired, sprinkle the top with chia seeds and cinnamon.

Chocolate-Dipped Strawberries

Ingredients:

1 pint fresh strawberries (about 12-15 strawberries)

4 oz dark chocolate (70% cocoa), chopped

1 tbsp coconut oil (optional, for smoother coating)

1/4 cup crushed nuts (optional, for garnish)

1/4 cup shredded coconut (optional, for garnish)

Prep Time: 15 minutes

Calories per Serving: 80 calories

Nutritional Information (per 2 strawberries):

Calories: 80

Protein: 1g

Carbohydrates: 10g

Sugars: 8g

Fat: 4g

Saturated Fat: 3g

Fiber: 2g

Instructions:

1. Prepare the strawberries by washing and thoroughly drying them, leaving the green stems on.

2. Melt Chocolate: Heat chopped dark chocolate and coconut oil (if using) in a microwave-safe basin for 30 seconds, stirring until smooth.

3. Dunk Strawberries: Holding each strawberry by its stem, dunk it into

the molten chocolate, coating about 3/4 of the berry.

4. Toppings: While the chocolate is still wet, sprinkle with crushed almonds or shredded coconut as desired.

5. Set Chocolate: Arrange dipped strawberries on a parchment-lined tray. Chill in the refrigerator for at least 15 minutes, or until chocolate has set. Serve immediately or refrigerate in an airtight container for up to three days.

Veggie Sticks with Guacamole

Ingredients:

For the Veggie Sticks:

2 large carrots, peeled and cut into sticks

2 celery stalks, trimmed and cut into sticks

1 red bell pepper, sliced into strips

1 cucumber, peeled and sliced into sticks

For the Guacamole:

2 ripe avocados

1 small lime, juiced

1 small tomato, diced

1/4 cup red onion, finely chopped

1 clove garlic, minced

1/4 cup fresh cilantro, chopped

Salt and pepper to taste

Prep Time: 15 minutes

Calories per Serving: 100 calories

Nutritional Information (per serving of guacamole with veggie sticks):

Fat: 8g

Carbohydrates: 10g

Protein: 2g

Fiber: 6g

Sugar: 3g

Instructions:

1. Prepare the vegetables: Wash and peel carrots and cucumbers. Cut carrots and celery into sticks, and cut the bell pepper and cucumber into strips.

2. Make the guacamole: Cut avocados in half, remove the pit, and scoop out the meat into a basin. Mash the avocados with a fork until smooth

yet slightly lumpy. Combine lime juice, diced tomato, red onion, garlic, and cilantro. Mix until thoroughly mixed. Season with salt and pepper to taste.

3. Serve: Arrange the vegetable sticks on a plate. Serve with a bowl of guacamole to dip.

Chia Pudding
Ingredients:

3 tablespoons chia seeds

1 cup unsweetened almond milk (or other low-calorie plant-based milk)

1 tablespoon honey or maple syrup (optional for sweetness)

1/2 teaspoon vanilla extract

Fresh berries or fruit for topping

Prep Time: 10 minutes (plus 2 hours of chilling)

Calories per Serving: 180 calories (without toppings)

Nutritional Information (per serving):

Protein: 5g

Fat: 10g

Carbohydrates: 15g

Fiber: 10g

Sugar: 5g (if using honey or syrup)

Instructions:

1. Ingredients: In a mixing bowl, combine chia seeds, almond milk, honey (if using), and vanilla essence.

2. Chill: Refrigerate for at least 2 hours or overnight. The chia seeds will absorb liquid and thicken.

3. Stir: Once chilled, stir the custard to break up any clumps. To serve, top with your favourite fresh berries or fruit.

Frozen Banana Bites

Ingredients:

2 large ripe bananas

1/2 cup dark chocolate chips (70% cocoa or higher)

1 tbsp coconut oil

1/4 cup chopped nuts (optional, for added crunch)

Pinch of sea salt (optional)

Prep Time: 10 minutes

Calories per Serving: 80 calories (per 2 bites)

Nutritional Information (per 2 bites):

Fat: 5g

Carbohydrates: 8g

Protein: 1g

Fiber: 1g

Sugar: 6g

Instructions:

1. Prepare bananas: Peel and slice bananas into half-inch rounds. Melt chocolate. In a microwave-safe bowl, combine the dark chocolate chips and coconut oil. Heat in 30-second intervals, swirling frequently, until melted and smooth.

2. Dip the bananas: Dip each banana slice into the melted chocolate, coating about half to three-quarters of it.

3. Add toppings: Sprinkle with chopped nuts and a pinch of sea salt, if desired.

4. Freeze: Place the dipped banana slices on a parchment-lined baking sheet. Freeze for at least an hour, or until the chocolate has set.

5. Serve: Enjoy directly from the freezer. Keep leftovers in an airtight jar in the freezer for up to two weeks.

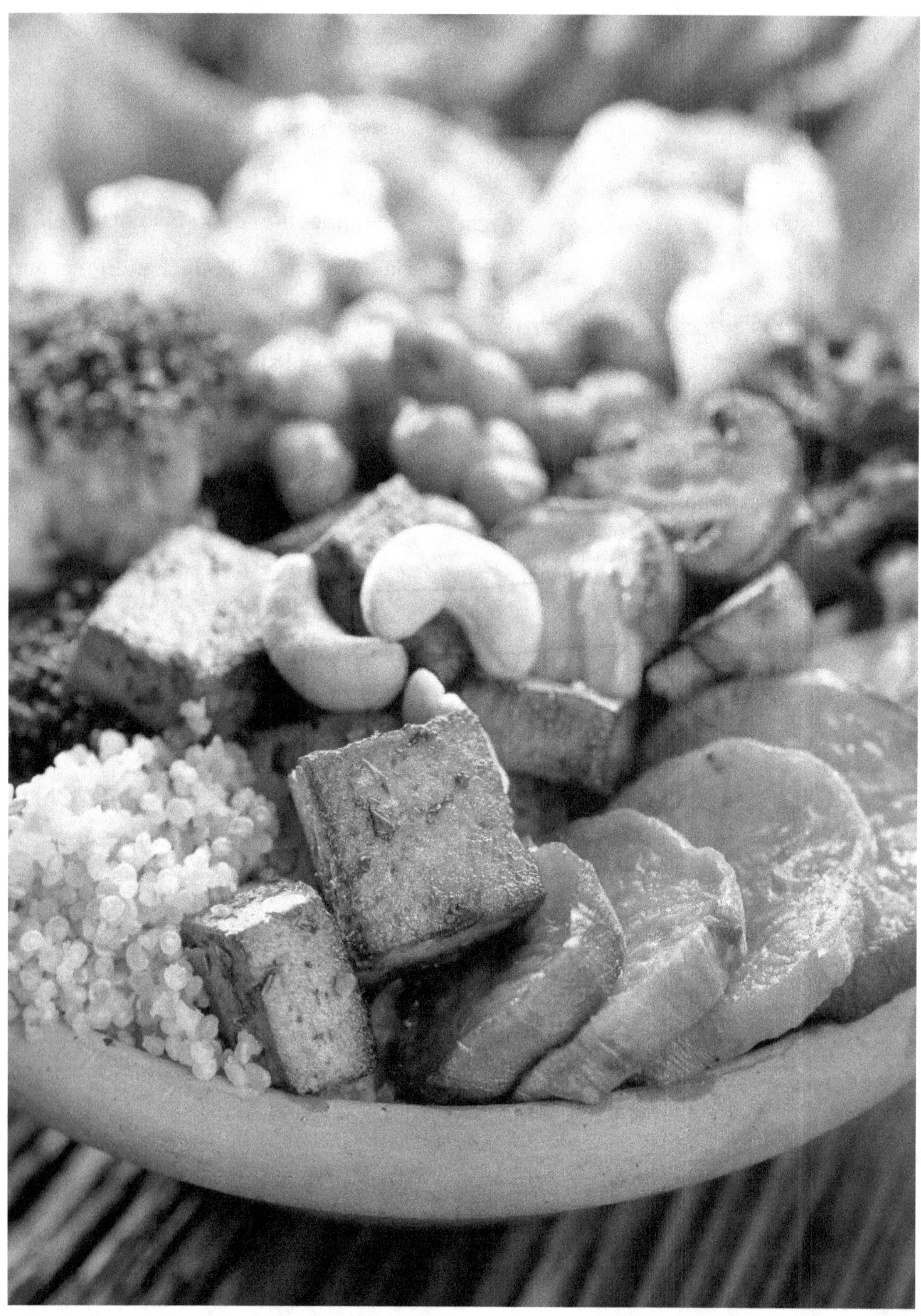